the
Origin
diet

the Origin diet

How Eating Like Our Stone Age Ancestors
Will Maximize Your Health

ELIZABETH SOMER, M.A., R.D.

Henry Holt and Company
New York

As only one link in an ancient human chain, I feel blessed to have come from such solid roots and to have the opportunity to pass on the best of what I've been given to generations to come. I dedicate this book to my family who stretch back beyond imaginable time and to my husband, Patrick, and my children, Lauren and William, their unborn children, and those generations to come who carry our legacy into the future.

Henry Holt and Company, LLC
Publishers since 1866
115 West 18th Street
New York, New York 10011

Henry Holt® is a registered trademark of
Henry Holt and Company, LLC.

Library of Congress Cataloging-in-Publication Data

Somer. Elizabeth.
   The origin diet: how eating like our stone age ancestors will maximize
your health / Elizabeth Somer.
      p.   cm.
   Includes bibliographical references and index.
   ISBN 0-8050-6335-8 (hb)
   1. Reducing diets.   2. Nutrition.   3. Weight loss.   4. Human
evolution.   I. Title.

RM222.2 .S6546 2001
613.2'5—dc21   00-056696

Henry Holt books are available for special
promotions and premiums. For details contact:
Director, Special Markets.

Designed by Paula Russell Szafranski

First Edition 2001

Printed in the United States of America

1   3   5   7   9   10   8   6   4   2

The nutritional and health information presented in this book is based on an in-depth review of the current scientific literature. It is intended only as an informative resource guide to help you make informed decisions; it is not meant to replace the advice of a physician or to serve as a guide to self-treatment. Always seek competent medical help for any health condition or if there is any question about the appropriateness of a procedure or health recommendation.

Contents

Acknowledgments

Just as our ancestors relied on the support of dear friends, family, and other clan members, so this endeavor is the product of my supportive tribe. A thousand thank-you's to my dearly loved family, Patrick, Lauren, and Will, for putting up with one more book deadline and for willingly tasting the recipes—both the successes and the failures; Jeanette Williams and Robin Vitetta for their gourmet palates and help with the recipes; Janet Haley, who faithfully read every word; David Smith, who is the best agent an author could ever hope to have; Martha Kaufman for tending the office, typing the reading list, and organizing the research and references; Miriam at Salem Public Library for, once again, searching around the nation for what must have seemed like hundreds of research articles; Victoria Dolby-Toews for another year of living at the medical library in search of research; Deb Brody, who inherited this project and loved it as if it were her own; and the staff at Henry Holt, who always make me feel so at home.

An extra-special thank-you to Dr. George Armelagos at Emory University, who took time out of his busy life to read chapters 1 and 2. Finally, I am grateful to all the people who have adopted the Origin Diet and been so willing to give me feedback, suggestions, and comments, especially the staff at both the Courthouse Athletic Club and In Shape in Salem, Oregon, and Natalie Baxter, Donnah Blalock, Katherine Ferrell, Richard Finicle, Amie Gallegoes, David and Patricia Hollenbeck, Sharon Johnston, Tim and Nicki Parrish, Emma Pfeiffer, Ernest and Linda Teal, Todd Washington, and Rollie and Dolores Wisbrock.

Although distant members of my tribe, I also want to thank all the researchers who took time to explain their research, including Tom Baranowski, Ph.D., at Baylor College of Medicine; Jeffrey Blumberg, Ph.D., at the USDA Human Nutrition Research Center on Aging at Tufts University; Kelly Brownell, Ph.D., at Yale University; C. Wayne Callaway, M.D., at George Washington University; Nancy Clark, M.S., R.D., at SportsMedicine Brookline; William Connor, M.D., at the Oregon Health Sciences University; Richard Coss, Ph.D., at the University of California, Davis; Winston Craig, Ph.D., R.D., at Andrews University; Bess Dawson-Hughes, Ph.D., at the USDA Human Nutrition Research Center on Aging at Tufts University; William Dietz, M.D., Ph.D., at the Centers for Disease Control and Prevention; Adam Drewnowski, Ph.D., at the University of Washington; S. Boyd Eaton, M.D., at Emory University; Sharon Edelstein, M.S., at George Washington University; Irvin Emanuel, M.D., at the University of Washington; Mary Enig, Ph.D., formerly at the University of Maryland; John Foreyt, Ph.D., at Baylor College of Medicine; Lauri Hager, Ph.D., at the University of California, Berkeley; Robert P. Heaney, M.D., at Creighton University; Susan Krebs-Smith, Ph.D., R.D., at the National Cancer Institute; Penny Kris-Etherton, Ph.D., R.D., at Pennsylvania State University; David Kritchevsky, Ph.D., at the University of Pennsylvania; Sarah Leibowitz, Ph.D., at Rockefeller University; Jane Leserman, Ph.D., at the University of North Carolina; Stephen Macko, Ph.D., at the University of Virginia; Mark Messina, Ph.D., at Loma Linda University; James Pennebaker, Ph.D., at the University of Texas; Ed Pierce, Ph.D., at the University of Richmond in Virginia; Barbara Rolls, Ph.D., at Pennsylvania State University; George Roth, M.D., at the National Institute on Aging; Robert Sack, Ph.D., at the Oregon Health Sciences University; Ellen Satter, R.D.; Evelyn Tribole, M.S., R.D.; Thomas Wadden, Ph.D., at the University of Pennsylvania; and Walter Willett, M.D., Dr. P.H., at the Harvard School of Public Health.

Introduction

You Were Born to Be Healthy,
Lean, and to Live Long

Nothing in biology makes sense except in light of evolution.
—THEODOSIUS DOBZHANSKY, 1973

Finally, it all made sense. I leaned back after reading an article on evolutionary nutrition and sighed in relief. My mind was racing with possibilities. So, before you bite into your next double cheeseburger or quench your thirst with a cola, I'd like a moment of your time. What I have to say will change your life!

I'm a research junkie. I read hundreds of studies every month and have done so for more than twenty years. As editor-in-chief of the newsletter *Nutrition Alert*, contributing editor to *Shape* magazine, and frequent correspondent for national news media, I pride myself on presenting accurate, timely nutrition information. From my thirty-two file drawers brimming with research, I can pull reams of studies that show vegetables lower cancer risk, saturated fat causes heart disease, fiber curbs appetite, calcium strengthens bones, or any other topic you desire. I have read the reports that obesity is on the rise and can describe in detail every theory to explain this epidemic. My files are jammed with research on how frailty associated with aging has more to do with sedentary living than with getting older, and that belonging to a support group can lower disease risks. I know the studies that formed the basis for the dietary guidelines and the Food Guide Pyramid. But, up until that one article, I had understood only the *whats* of nutrition. I was filled with a thousand *whys*:

- Why do vegetables lower cancer risk?
- Why does saturated fat accumulate in arteries, blocking blood flow, and leading to heart disease, while fish oils lower our risk?
- Why do our bodies absorb only 10 percent of the iron in our diets (which places up to 80 percent of women during the childbearing years at risk for iron deficiency), but up to 95 percent of the fat?
- Why does our risk for many diseases, from cancer to cataracts, increase as we age?
- Why do we gain weight when our bodies are so perfectly designed to be fit?

The article on evolutionary nutrition explained the *whys* simply and clearly. It was an "Ah-ha" moment when decades of research fell into place. It began my quest to know more. The end result is this book.

Hello Grandpa!

Still haven't touched that cheeseburger or cola? Good. Now stop for a moment and think back. I mean *way* back. Neither of these foods, or any processed food for that matter, ever graced the lips of even one of our ancient ancestors, dating back tens of thousands of generations.

For 99 percent of the time humans have been on earth, our ancestors ate and evolved on diets of plants and very lean wild game. These diets served our ancestors well. In fact, our Paleolithic grandparents lived free of heart disease, cancer, diabetes, hypertension, osteoporosis, cataracts, and other modern diseases. They also remained lean and strong throughout life. The most fit, the smartest, and the strongest lived to pass on their genes from one generation to the next like an unbroken chain. Today, that nutritional legacy lives in us.

Agriculture developed about ten thousand years ago, followed later by the Industrial Revolution. These two events brought cataclysmic changes to our dining habits, converting us from hunters and gatherers to farmers, then to drivers of cars with automatic gears and power steering. These last few thousand years are only a minute in evolutionary time, accounting for little or no change in our biological makeup.

Therein lies the problem. It takes tens of thousands of years for the body to adapt to even small changes in the environment. Our biochemistry and physiology remain fine-tuned to diets and activity levels that existed tens of thousands of years ago. Escalating obesity and disease rates are just some of the results when genetics collides with lifestyle. In essence, we remain cave dwellers dressed in designer jeans, genetically programmed to thrive on a diet of nuts, seeds, leaves, honey, and wild game, but gorging on doughnuts, cheese puffs, domesticated beef, soda pop . . . well, you get the picture.

The more I researched the anthropological and archeological data, the more my years of nutrition research fell into place. We don't need vegetables just because they're good for us. It's when we *don't* supply the body with the fuels and building blocks it needs that the system breaks down, just as our cars would stall if we were to pour sand or grease into their fuel tanks. Our diets today are killing us because they are as alien to our bodies as breathing in carbon monoxide! Suddenly, it all made sense. If we returned to our dietary roots (and tubers) and ate in balance with our evolutionary makeup, we'd live in harmony with our bodies, experience an extraordinary state of good health, and sidestep just about every chronic disease, as well as maintain a healthy weight and live longer!

My Six Promises

My background in nutrition gave me the edge when reading the hundreds of studies on archeology and anthropology that went into researching this book. I know how to decipher this information in light of today's nutritional needs and lifestyles. I also knew how to glean the best research that would give the most thorough and accurate account of what our bodies need, both in light of evolution as well as in today's modern world. What I learned was:

When we eat and move in balance with the way our bodies evolved, we do much more than just avoid disease. We achieve a level of health and vitality that many of us have never before experienced. That level of health is not only possible, it's embedded in our cells. It's our inherent biological right.

Don't worry. You don't have to live in a cave, hunt woolly mammoths, or eat only wild greens and roots to achieve these goals. You can still have your favorite recipes, eat in restaurants, and order takeout. On the other hand, the Origin Diet in this book will ask you to consider giving up (or at least cutting back on) foods like bacon, soda pop, and cream (not common items on a Stone Age plate!).

The rewards are worth it. Adopt even a few suggestions in the Origin Diet and I guarantee you'll feel better within weeks. Practice most of the guidelines and you will see noticeable changes in your weight and disease risk, such as lowering of blood cholesterol levels. Take on the entire program and you'll experience significant improvements in how you feel, think, and live. You might even reverse the damage already done by past poor eating habits, turning back the clock on numerous diseases, such as atherosclerosis and bone loss. All because you'll be fueling your body with the foods on which it thrives.

This is much more than a hope. It is a promise. Live by the Five Stone Age Secrets and follow the advice in the Original Dozen discussed in this book, and I promise

1. you will reduce your risk for all major age-related diseases, including heart disease, diabetes, hypertension, cancer, osteoporosis, cataracts, and even depression;
2. you will think more clearly, including having better memory throughout life;
3. you will stack the deck in favor of living longer and spending those extra years healthier;
4. you will lose weight and keep the weight off;

5. you will have more energy; and

6. you will enjoy life more.

A Tried-and-True Plan

Those aren't empty promises. Many people have taken me up on the challenge and found that the results are even better than they imagined. People who have adopted the Origin Diet and Workout Program in this book have lost weight (up to thirty pounds in fifteen weeks!), lowered their risks for heart disease (including dramatic reductions in blood cholesterol levels and blood pressure), increased their energy, found they slept better, had fewer cravings for sweets, experienced improvements in mood, and even reduced medications. It makes sense. Reconnect with your body's ancient heritage, fuel your body in harmony with your evolutionary roots, and you will maximize your health, energy, and mental ability.

We influence our destinies by the foods we eat. You can sidestep disease, boost your energy, maintain your mental clarity, lose unwanted extra pounds, live longer, and enjoy life more if you return to a style of eating more closely attuned to the natural needs of your body. You'll find out how in the following chapters. Enjoy your journey back to the future!

PART I

■ ■ ■

Sizing Up Our Designer Genes

1

A Look at the Family Album

You are what you eat.

You've heard that adage a million times. You've probably even experienced it when you skip breakfast only to battle midafternoon fatigue. Or when you've seen someone eat a high-fat diet over a lifetime only to end up with heart disease in later years. But the link between food and you goes much deeper.

For example, you are what your mother ate. Inadequate nutrition during pregnancy increases the infant's risk later in life for heart disease, high blood pressure, glucose intolerance and diabetes, reduced intellectual ability, impaired immunity, and even obesity. According to Irvin Emanuel, M.D., professor of epidemiology and pediatrics at the University of Washington in Seattle, the nutritional status of our grandmothers and great-grandmothers affects our health by influencing how well our mothers and their mothers developed in the womb.

The connection goes even further, extending back millions of years to the roots of the human race and beyond. Nutrition has always been a primary driving force shaping who we are as a species—from our brain size and height, sweat glands, and our famous opposable thumbs to the enzymes that break down foods for digestion, the nerve chemicals that affect our appetites and moods, and the hormones that regulate our daily and monthly cycles. Even our ability to communicate and cooperate and the development of societies are by-products of the foods we ate then and now. You inherited your blue or brown eyes from your parents (which they inherited from their parents and so on), but the fact that you have eyes that see is a consequence of the right nutrients, such as vitamin A, being in the right place at the right time millions of years ago to allow the evolution of sight.

There are evolutionary reasons for every aspect of why we are so intricately intertwined with food, including why

- we are one of the few species unable to make vitamin C;
- we absorb only about 10 percent of the iron, but 95 percent of the fat we consume;
- saturated fat is a dietary poison to our bodies;
- we crave chocolate, not beet greens; and
- our brains require amounts of certain fats and antioxidants that are difficult to obtain from modern diets. (These and other topics will be discussed in subsequent chapters.)

The human body is a product of the nutrients available over the course of hundreds of millions of years. No matter how excellent the architect's plans, the building (our bodies) would never have been built without the necessary materials. Since food provides the fundamental materials that determined how we evolved, you literally are what you, your parents, grandparents, and every ancestor before that ate.

Each generation has contributed to our gradual evolution from simple one-celled organisms to plants to furry critters, and finally in the past several million years to primates and now to our current selves—known formally as *Homo sapiens sapiens* (meaning "doubly wise"). Our lineage survived because each generation consumed the right mix of nutrients that allowed future generations to evolve. Only the strongest, the most adapted to their environments, the most agile, intelligent, swift, and healthy made it. That's how natural selection works. It sculpted our species, in large part by the nutrients available and eaten by our ancient ancestors. Just as mother's milk is uniquely tailored to an infant's needs, so our evolutionary diets were the nutritional equivalent to mother's milk for our evolving bodies.

What were those diets like? On what foods did our bodies evolve, thrive, develop, and ultimately populate the planet? More importantly, what do those ancient diets have to do with our daily lives, our mental and physical health, and even the aging process? Since the past is always a useful key to the future, here's a bird's-eye look at our ancient ancestors' dinner tables and how a few recent changes to the plate have turned our health upside down.

From Swamp to Savanna

Thank heaven for algae! Given 3 billion years, this slime oxygenated the planet, allowing plants to grow. A few million years after plants arrived, animals evolved and crept out of the blue-green swamps onto the land. About 75 million years ago, after the forests had spread over the planet, insect-eating mammals roamed the land. They had evolved on diets rich in special fats called omega-3 fatty acids made from algae. Their nervous systems and vision had developed as a result of ample amounts of these fats and of beta carotene, which was converted to retinol to be used as the receptor in the eyes for vision. About 55 million years ago a shrew-like critter climbed into a tree searching for tasty bugs. The food was good and predators were few, so he and his friends stayed in the trees.

It was a primate "life of Riley" in the forest canopy for our earliest ancestors, with each lineage evolving as a result of the foods they ate. They lost their claws and developed grasping hands with nails so they could handle delicate seeds. Future generations developed depth perception and the ability to see colors, which gave them an edge when searching for fruit and escaping predators.

At some point, a curious tree lover ventured to the ground, perhaps in search of fallen fruit. Maybe the forests were shrinking and he or she ran out of food in the trees. Or perhaps that tree lover, having put on a little too much weight, simply broke the branch beneath his or her feet and fell to earth. Thus began life on the ground for the primate family.

About 3.75 to 3.2 million years ago, a descendant of the tree lovers, a humanlike creature called *Australopithecus afarensis,* became an expert at exploiting the earthly environment (the well-known "Lucy" found in the Hadar region of Ethiopia was of this species). Although more ape-like than human, *A. afarensis* walked upright and expanded the traditional diet of fruits and leaves to include grasses and protein-rich bugs and possibly small animals. The diet was rich in vitamin E, protein, omega-3 fatty acids, and carotenes, such as beta carotene. *A. afarensis* is suspected to be the first in a line of known ancestors leading to modern-day humans. Although other lineages would sprout from this common ancestor, such as *Australopithecus robustus,* they would die out, possibly because of limited or poor food choices. Dietary variety had become essential for survival.

The age-old advice to eat a variety of foods is actually based on habits developed over several million years and was the secret to our ultra-great-grandparents' evolutionary success. Their high-quality diets were based on a wide array of foods (up to 333 different species of plants, insects, and small animals) and were richer in protein and high-calorie foods than diets of previous generations. Our ancestors had developed digestive tracts that allowed maximum absorption of calories, fats, proteins, and nutrients. The extra calories allowed the dietary flexibility essential to survival during times of severe climate change. The special fats provided the structural components for a more complex brain and better vision. The antioxidant-rich plants helped these humanlike critters maintain a vigorous immune system and provided optimal protection of tissues against the toxic oxygen fragments that we now call free radicals. While the big jump in brain size wouldn't happen for another million or so years, this was the beginning. In contrast, the children of both the tree lovers and *Australopithecus africanus* who stuck with their limited diet of leaves and fruits evolved into modern-day mammals such as the lemur, gorilla, or gibbon, or became extinct.

THE FIRST HANDY MAN

About 2 to 2.5 million years ago, a new descendant appeared on the African scene, the first member of our genus, *Homo habilis* (meaning "handy man"). He is considered the first toolmaker, crafting primitive scrapers and blades to cut meat from the bones of scavenged animals at Olduvai Gorge and elsewhere in Africa. Then, about 1.8 to 1.6 million years ago, *Homo erectus* (also called Java Man) was born.

H. erectus was more robust than we, but like us expended up to three times more calories to maintain a larger brain than any other previous primate. Up to 25 percent of all calories went to brain function (in contrast, monkeys use only about 8 percent of their calories to fuel brain power). This meant that *H. erectus* creatures had to beef up their diets. While they may have courageously attacked and slaughtered large wild game, it's just as likely they sneaked out of the bushes to scavenge bits and pieces of a competitor's kill.

What's important is they were humanlike. They used weapons and tools, such as crude hand axes. Their ability to walk and run for miles allowed them to actively and purposefully search for food throughout a wide area. They kept the campfires burning to prepare food and possibly drive game toward killing sites. They also liked meat in amounts unheard of for the rest of the primate family. They were well on their way to developing a division of labor where women gathered roots, fruit, honey, leaves, pistachios, almonds, wild figs, acorns, grass seeds and grains, beans, and other wild plants, while men spent time hunting or scavenging for meat. This teamwork approach to food gathering led to the most diverse diet of any primate that had ever walked the earth. It was also the highest quality diet of any animal on the planet. These dietary choices were so successful that all of our ancestors from that time on would be hunter-gatherers.

Somewhere between 500,000 and 180,000 years ago, the first *Homo sapiens* appeared on earth and gradually replaced *H. erectus*. Called archaic *Homo sapiens,* they lived side by side with another humanlike neighbor—*Homo neanderthalensis* (alias the Neanderthals, named for the Neander Valley in Germany where their remains were first found). By this time, our ancestors were quite adept at getting along. Their survival depended on their large brains, which could maintain a mental map of plant food supplies, knowledge of how to get to the food, and complex relationships with fellow tribesmen in cooperating and communicating who would chase the rabbit and who would catch it.

WHY MEAT?

Why was meat so important to our evolutionary progress? The brain is an expensive organ to maintain, so natural selection wouldn't have favored it unless a larger brain gave our ancestors some kind of advantage, such as in helping them find better foods and stay out of harm's way. Meat is the only food packed with enough fat and calories to supply the necessary extra energy for our ancestors' expanding brains. The diet-brain link created a domino effect that worked in our favor. Adding meat to the diet allowed the brains of *H. erectus* to increase in size and complexity. *H. erectus* then used his brain power to solve diet problems, which helped his descendants develop still bigger brains. He was so successful that his lineage survived until 300,000 years ago, outliving all other humanlike species that had roamed the planet until that time.

Much as we navigate the aisles of our local supermarket, knowing where to find the cereal, the canned peaches, or the fresh spinach, the first *H. sapiens* knew their supermarket well, only it was two to three miles across and they lived in it. They took mental stock of where and when to harvest wild roots, what types of trees produced the best fruit, and where the fox holes could be found. They navigated their complex world using their increasingly more thoughtful and creative brains.

Archaic *H. sapiens* also lived in communities and brought their food back to camp rather than eat it on the spot, something no other primate had ever done. They bartered and shared their food. None of these social skills would have been possible if not for their mixed diets of roots, leaves, nuts, honey, grass seeds and grains, beans, vegetables, and meat, which provided the right combination of fuel and nutrients to build better brains and more adept bodies.

TALL, LEAN, AND SMART

Archeologists have found thousands of skeletal and campsite remains of the people who walked the earth 180,000 years ago. These people were pretty much like us. They quickly spread from Africa to the rest of the world. They lived side by side with Neanderthals in Europe until about 30,000 years ago, when their hairier, more robust neighbors became extinct. This left our direct ancestors alone for the first time in history, the only remaining descendants of all previous humanlike creatures.

By 40,000 years ago (an era called the Upper Paleolithic in Europe and the Stone Age period in Africa), *Homo sapiens sapiens* (that's us) had populated the earth. Dress them in suits and ties or little black dresses and heels and they'd look like everyone else on the street today, maybe better. Their limbs were leaner and more agile than those of any of their predecessors. They were slightly taller than we—the men averaged 5' 10" and the women were at least 5' 6"—and they had beautiful smiles (only 2 percent of the fossil teeth show any sign of tooth decay).

Within a few thousand years, our Paleolithic grandparents had progressed more than *Homo erectus* and his archaic *sapiens* successors had in the previous million years. Our Paleolithic ancestors invented tools, such as blades made from bone, ivory, and antlers, to make boats, spears, harpoons, snares, fish hooks, snowshoes, and probably bows and arrows. With this stockpile of weaponry, it's no wonder they were skilled hunters of big game. They used highly sophisticated hunting strategies that required planning and teamwork, such as driving game through narrow bottlenecks where the game would be ambushed. In line with their heritage, they complemented their meat intake with an abundance of leaves, roots, stalks, mushrooms, fruits, berries, tubers, and other plants.

Food was abundant and life was good for our Paleolithic grandparents. They worked hard, but had ample time for leisure activities. During their extended "weekends," they became artists, painting caves with some of the world's finest pictures. They made elaborate jewelry to adorn their bodies. They sculpted flutes, played music, and danced at parties where a wealth of traditional foods were served fresh, raw, roasted, steamed, and boiled.

The Tree of Life

Many branches of the evolutionary tree are yet to be identified and it is likely that the tree is more like a bush, with many kinds of humanlike species having lived simultaneously. The known fossil record looks something like the scheme below, with our species—*Homo sapiens sapiens*—having evolved over millions of years from ancestors such as *Australopithecus afarensis*.

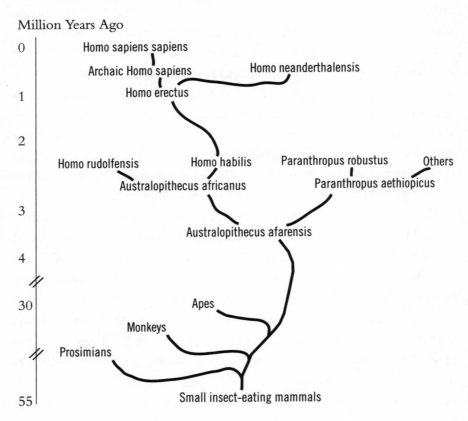

Million Years Ago

Their lives centered around family and community. They lived in small communities that bartered with close-knit systems of neighboring tribes. They formed political alliances, developed medicines and rituals for healing, formed complex languages, buried their dead with elaborate ceremony, and celebrated the seasons. They were the first philosophers, contemplating the world, not just the moment, creating symbols and images for unexplainable beliefs, and formulating insights. The elders were honored for their wisdom, the children probably sat around the campfire at night to hear stories. The written word was yet to be invented, but parents passed down their family memories from generation to generation through rich and colorful stories and fables.

If each and every one of us could trace our family lineage back far enough, say about two thousand generations, we would all find a Paleolithic grandparent who lived this ancient yet sophisticated hunter-gatherer life. These people were more than an improved version of their ancestry, they were a giant leap unprecedented in the history of the world. Yet it was their ancestors who had set the stage for their development, and it is their biology that we carry within us today.

Our Paleolithic grandparents were the culmination of an unbroken, evolving chain of millions of generations of hunters and gatherers. They were in perfect balance with their environment. Their bodies, like those of all their ancestors, thrived like no other humanlike creature because they ate a wide variety of plants and animals. Even compared to their next-door neighbors the Neanderthals, who died young from trauma and malnutrition, the people of the Upper Paleolithic period were as strong as any athletes today, and when they survived the common killers of the day—infection, accidents, and childbirth—lived robustly into their sixties and beyond. All this changed about ten thousand years ago (called the Neolithic period or New Stone Age) when our ancestors switched from foraging to farming.

From Forests to Fields

No one is quite sure why our ancestors put down the hand ax and took up the plow. Perhaps the lush landscape of the post–Ice Age era with its wealth of rich grasses made it easy to cultivate a few hardy seeds. Or perhaps enough wild game had been killed or hunted to extinction that these ancient people were forced to look for alternative food sources.

The first experiments were probably nothing more than just expanding the strains of wild plants by broadcasting some of the harvested seed over a wider area. Our ancestors would have learned quickly that the harvest from this first crop could be stored, which curbed hunger during the winter months. After eons of hunting wild game and plants, it must have been a discovery worthy of the Nobel Prize—by developing more elaborate ways to prepare the soil, weed, till, and cultivate hardy food, people could have a dependable source of food. For the first time in their history they settled down, relaxed a little, and were assured there was a more predictable food supply to get them through the winter.

Somewhere between 4,500 and 10,000 years ago, hunter-gatherer societies in at least seven different regions of the world independently domesticated plants and made wild animals their pets and livestock.* The prospects of farming were so enticing that within two to three centuries or about four to six generations (keep in mind that evolution up until this point had been measured in hundreds of thousands and millions of years), people in any one geographical region had domesticated three of the seven core grains. Agriculture had initiated a turning point in the long evolutionary history of our species equal in magnitude to the impact of an asteroid. If our ancient ancestors had known what this radical change would bring, they might not have been so quick to abandon their age-old lifestyles.

Far from the glorious ascent into civilization, the shift from a hunter-gatherer life to farming brought health problems never before experienced by any species. The hunter-gatherer diet had been highly diversified, rich in thousands of wild foods, and supplied about 30 to 35 percent of its nutrients from animals and the remaining 65 to 70 percent from Mother Nature's richest plants. In the blink of an evolutionary eye, people became less physically active and ate more of less-varied diets. Of the 50,000 to 100,000 edible plants on the planet, only 3,000 were kept for food, and of these only 150 were cultivated; no edible plants have

---

*Domestication is the human creation of a new form of animal or plant, one that is distinctly different from its wild predecessor or living wild relatives.

been added to that list in thousands of years. Today, the people of the world live on fewer than 20 main crops. "Once people subsisted on farming, rather than the diversified food supply obtained from hunting and gathering, they depended more and more on staples like maize and wheat, which upset the balance and diversity of the food supply," says George Armelagos, Ph.D., professor of anthropology at Emory University in Atlanta and coauthor of *Consuming Passions: The Anthropology of Eating*.

Granted, agriculture resulted in greater yields of food per acre than our Paleolithic ancestors experienced. The irony is that with more food came malnutrition. The domesticated animals (such as wild sheep, pigs, and goats) and plants (especially barley and wild wheat) were not chosen because they were the most nutritious, but because they were the easiest to herd, store, and harvest. "The Paleolithic hunter-gatherer life was no Club Med, but these people at least got a variety of foods by tapping into native food resources in their environment. Agriculture put an end to variety, creating superfoods of a few grains, such as maize," says Dr. Armelagos.

Because there was no understanding of how diet affects health, nutrient deficiencies became the plague of most households:

- Bodies accustomed to a wide variety of foods rich in vitamin A developed blindness and skin conditions as people ate fewer dark green vegetables and liver.
- Beriberi, pellagra, and other B vitamin–deficiency diseases developed and persisted into the 1800s.
- Protein and mineral deficiencies became common and continued into the twentieth century.
- Compromised nutritional status suppressed immune systems, which were accustomed to higher-nutrient diets. Combined with living in close proximity, this left people defenseless against a barrage of infectious diseases, including typhus, sleeping sickness, smallpox, and measles, the latter having originated as a disease of domesticated animals that adapted to humans. Schistosomiasis (a parasitic infection

caused by a species of fluke, whose symptoms include pain, organ dysfunction, and anemia) was a problem for those farmers standing thigh-deep in contaminated watery canals. Milk from infected cattle transmitted tuberculosis. Wool and skins were infected with anthrax. Rats, mice, and sparrows exposed people to bubonic plague and rabies. Poor sanitation, crowded living conditions, and increased consumption of old or spoiled food only aggravated the problem.

- Tooth decay and loss, anemia, osteoporosis, poor wound healing, and poor skeletal growth in children were new health problems.
- Height, a standard indicator of nutritional status, dropped four to six inches and would not return to Paleolithic levels until the latter part of the twentieth century.
- Brain size began to decrease; today the human brain is approximately 11 percent smaller than it was prior to agriculture.

In hunter-gatherer groups, food is shared with neighbors. As a result, everyone benefits from what their tribe gathers or hunts, and young and old are fed alike. In contrast, the rise of agriculture resulted in a net loss of general well-being for everyone except those owning land or possessions—the rich.

"Agriculture took the highest toll on women and children," says Dr. Armelagos. Our Paleolithic ancestors unknowingly spaced their babies, so women's bodies had time to recuperate from pregnancy. Their children were nursed for years, which offset the danger of malnutrition during critical growth years. Agriculture created a demand for labor that was met by increasing family size, weaning children early, and shortening time between pregnancies. The nutritional status of women and children suffered. Infant mortality increased, and malformed pelvises from inadequate intake of calcium were so common in women that a German physician named M. O. Prochownick in the 1880s advocated a fluid-restricted, low-calorie diet during pregnancy to retard infant growth, which increased risks for the infant, but made childbirth easier for women with contracted pelvic bones. Rickets, characterized by bowed legs, was a common sign of vitamin D deficiency. Life expectancies for people living in ancient Rome to the beginning of the twentieth century seldom climbed above forty-nine years.

The social snowball unleashed by farming turned villages into towns, towns into city-states, and city-states into nations. Cities gained control of expanding agricultural lands, while empires and armies developed to protect claimed property. Soon there was no turning back. People congregated around agriculture as much from necessity as by choice. As opposed to their ancestors, who moved with the food and always left game and plants behind, farmers settled in permanent camps and depleted the local area of wild foods, either by killing, overharvesting, or destroying the natural habitat. This only made people more dependent on their cultivated crops and domesticated animals. The remaining hunter-gatherers were forced to take up the plow to survive. The population explosion started, with cities swelling to populations of 50,000 by 3000 B.C. Then, about two hundred years ago, something happened that further widened the gap between us and our evolutionary roots.

From Fields to Fast Foods

The steam engine invented by Thomas Newcomen in 1705 paved the way for the Industrial Revolution in the late eighteenth and early nineteenth centuries. Our ancestors' lives would change more in the next few years than in all of the ten thousand years before. William Shakespeare would be more bewildered by life in the twenty-first century than would an archaic *Homo sapiens* catapulted 290,000 years into the future to visit a hunter-gatherer tribe the year before the discovery of agriculture.

The legacy of the Industrial Revolution is that our most recent ancestors moved less and ate more processed foods. Today, machines do our work, we sit rather than hunt or gather and depend on cars instead of legs. Only within our grandparents' lifetimes has physical activity plummeted so drastically. The mechanization of farming alone dropped energy expenditure by 50 percent. Between 1956 and 1990, labor-saving devices cut calorie output by 65 percent. It's only a matter of decades since a sedentary lifestyle was defined as one where a person was intensely active for less than three hours daily. Now we applaud if we fit in physical activity for a half hour, three days a week.

Today's foods would not be recognized by the Pilgrims, let alone by our ancient ancestors. Our ancient grandparents preserved food by sun drying, oven drying, smoking, fermenting, and sometimes freezing. Foods today are spray-dried, extruded, microwaved, dehydrated, puffed, fortified, freeze-dried, reconstituted, hydrogenated, textured, irradiated, and more. Processing has turned low-calorie, nutrient-rich foods into low-nutrient, calorie-rich foods. While the first farmers merely cultivated wild grains, now brand names thrive on inventing different ways to package the starchy innards (the endosperms) of a few grains, which are virtually devoid of the nutrients and fiber found in the whole grain. This starch is mixed with fats, sugars, and salt at levels unprecedented in the history of our species.

Between 1900 and 1976 alone, fat consumption rose by 25 percent, with most coming from saturated fat. Instead of wild roots, we chomp on potato chips. We skip the wild rice and reach for the puffed rice. We choose strawberry jam, not strawberries. We quench our thirst with sweetened, caffeinated chemical brews, not mountain spring water. We prefer French fries to spinach, hot dogs to legumes, and fruit-flavored candy to cantaloupe. Refined grains are staples, not novelties; meat is domesticated, not wild; and vegetables, if eaten at all, are a side dish, not the main course.

Then there is the issue of variety. Today's global population relies on fewer than twenty staples, including wheat, maize, rice, barley, and oats. Potatoes are the only staple root crop, compared to the thousands of roots, grains, grass seeds, nuts, leafy plants, fruits, stalks, tubers, gums, and flowers that were staples in our ancient ancestors' diets. We eat a handful of domesticated meats, gobbling 12,000 hamburgers across the United States every minute, compared to the hundreds of species of wild game in our ancestors' diets. "Dietary variety no longer means how many different plants you eat, but rather how many different ways you can eat refined wheat or corn," says Dr. Armelagos. Food technologists are today's alchemists, transforming one grass seed—wheat—into more than 1,500 foods, from cookies, crackers, breads, and doughnuts to noodles, cereals, pancakes, and dumplings.

Now and Then: Fiber and Sugar Intakes

Compare our intakes of fiber and sugar with those of our ancient hunter-gatherer grandparents and you'll find little in common.

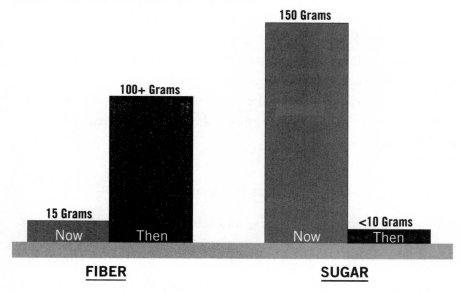

After millions of years of satisfying our sweet tooth with an occasional lick of honey, today we're dumping between twenty-nine and forty teaspoons of refined sugar onto our daily plates, which is radically different from even our grandparents' intakes, which were closer to four teaspoons at the turn of the twentieth century. Sugar is not just in candy, cakes, and desserts; it's also in baked beans, catsup, fruited yogurts, granola bars, and cereals, to name only a few. It's no wonder that only 2 percent of Paleolithics had teeth that were decayed, compared to 60 percent of those in the nineteenth century, and 95 percent of people today.

Even our pattern of eating has changed. Foragers for thousands of years nibbled, grazed, and snacked on mini-meals, with only an occasional feast when hunters brought back large game from a kill. When food was scarce, our ancestors fasted. Today, we depend on the three square meals a day, and our problem is too much, not too little, food all year around. (See chapter 4 for more on how our diets contribute to weight gain.)

We have traveled the equivalent of light years in the past few thousand years. Prior to ten thousand years ago, 100 percent of the 5 to 10 million humans on earth were hunter-gatherers. Slightly more than eight thousand years of farming brought the population up to 350 million, with only 1 percent being hunter-gatherers. Today, with the world bulging at 6 billion people, only a few thousand hunter-gatherers are left. Nutrition shaped the very essence of our lives, yet in the blink of an evolutionary eye, we radically altered our food, lives, and environments, so that today we are consuming foods as alien to our ancient bodies as breathing carbon monoxide.

Cave Dwellers in Designer Jeans

"For 100,000 generations people had been hunters and gatherers. Compare that to the 500 generations people have been farmers, the 10 generations since the Industrial Age, and the one generation since computers and you see that there have been major changes in how we live and eat in a very short period of time," says S. Boyd Eaton, M.D., adjunct associate professor of anthropology at Emory University in Atlanta. Never in the past 4 billion years has any animal, let alone any primate and certainly any human, eaten such an unnatural diet.

It takes tens of thousands of years for the body to adapt to even small changes in the environment, yet our lives have changed beyond recognition in only a few thousand years and cataclysmically in the past two hundred years. Our biochemistry and physiology have not caught up, so they remain fine-tuned to diets and activity levels that existed prior to ten thousand years ago. In essence, we are cave dwellers dressed in designer jeans. We might have switched from the hand ax to the food processor, but we remain genetically programmed to thrive on diets of nuts, seeds, leaves, honey, and wild game, while gorging on doughnuts, cheese puffs, domesticated beef, soda pop . . . well, you get the picture.

Keep in mind that the diet on which our ancient ancestors evolved for 99.8 percent of their time on earth was astonishingly successful, allowing our species to outlast all other humanlike creatures, evolving and eventually populating the entire planet. It's not by chance that we require carbohydrate-rich foods as our immediate source of energy, dietary fat for long-term fuel, or protein to build and repair muscles, organs, and tissues. We inherited those food requirements over millions of years, just as our bodies evolved on a specific level and diversity of nutrients that are no longer supplied by our current diets.

When Genes and Habits Collide

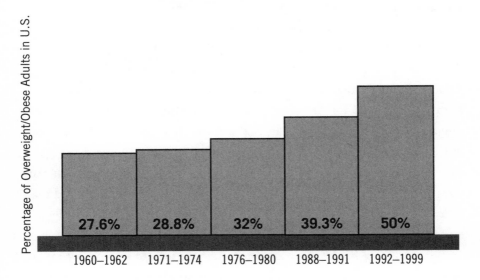

Compared to hunter-gatherer populations where obesity is rare or nonexistent, more Americans are getting fatter every year.

The results of this alien lifestyle surround us. Escalating obesity and chronic disease are some of the results of the collision between genetics and lifestyle. "Our ancestors who stored body fat efficiently resisted starvation during famines and lived to reproduce," says Dr. Armelagos. "Our bodies weren't designed for today's never-ending abundance of easily digested carbohydrates and fat, along with no activity."

Our Out-of-Sync Lifestyles

With this brief glance at our evolutionary makeup, it becomes clear how the statement "You are what you eat" is truly a prescription for who we are and from where we've come. We are products of what our ancestors ate as surely as we thrive on the same oxygen first released by algae billions of years ago. We're dying as a result of eating these current diets, just as we die when forced to breathe only carbon monoxide.

Our evolutionary diets over the course of millions of years produced a human body that is meant to be lean, fit, strong, resistant to infection, able to run and walk long distances, and to think fast and creatively throughout life. Most of our genes are of far greater antiquity than even the Paleolithic period, let alone since the development of agriculture. That same body that suited us so well for millions of years now finds itself ill-equipped for the diets of today, buckling under the pressure of our high-fat meals and low physical activity. It might sound ridiculous, but if we had evolved on today's lifestyles—watching spectator sports and television, eating highly processed junk food, and living with constant stress—the modern human would thrive on saturated fat and inactivity, succumbing to disease only when fed too many vegetables and forced to be physically active.

Granted, our Stone Age ancestors had health problems, which we would face today if not for advancements in sanitation, medicine, science, and safety standards. We no longer fear being attacked by a tiger while sleeping in caves, suffering with untreatable parasitic infections, or falling from a cliff while trying to spear a bison. We also have reasons to be thankful. Today our average life expectancy is more than seventy-five years, double that of preindustrial times. Infant death rates are lower than ever, and 80 percent of the babies born today can expect to live to retirement age.

Much of this improvement in life quality comes as a result of recent discoveries. By the middle of the last century, most of the vitamins had been discovered and enrichment of processed grains helped lower, but not eliminate, the risk of common nutrient diseases that had plagued people since the development of agriculture, including pellagra, beriberi, and anemia. Iodine was added to salt to prevent goiter, vitamin D was added to milk to prevent rickets, and recently folic acid was added to grains to help prevent birth defects, heart disease, and possibly cancer. We have learned much about how to fill in the nutritional gaps created by agriculture. With those kinds of health statistics and advancements in nutritional science, it might seem ridiculous to propose that we are ill-adapted to modern life. Yet an abundance of research shows our current diets and lifestyles are killing us, contributing to more than three out of every four deaths in this country alone.

The diseases of civilization—from heart disease, hypertension, and diabetes to cataracts, osteoporosis, and cancer—were apparently unknown to our ancient ancestors. The only chronic disease they faced in appreciable amounts was arthritis. Chronic disease is not the inevitable consequence of aging, but rather is the inevitable consequence of living out of sync with our evolutionary origins. For example,

- 70 percent of cancers are related to diet and lifestyle;
- 50 percent or more of heart disease is related to diet;
- middle-age spread is not related to age, it's related to activity; and
- frailty, feebleness, and disability are not natural consequences of aging, but the result of inactivity.

Of course, not everyone is enamored with the idea that our Stone Age ancestors were all that healthy. "Sure, Stone Age people didn't die of our diseases, but that's because they didn't live long enough," says David Kritchevsky, Ph.D., institute scholar, Wistar Institute, and professor of biochemistry at the University of Pennsylvania. "It's a huge step to compare our diets with theirs when the two lifestyles are so completely different."

But even when you compare modern-day hunter-gatherer populations (such as the !Kung San in southern Africa or the Ache in Paraguay) or even vegetarians who eat lots of fruits and vegetables, you get the same results. These people seldom develop heart disease, hypertension, diabetes, stroke, or all sorts of cancers. People who eat diets more akin to our origins also maintain desirable weights, live longer, think more clearly, have lower rates of depression and suicide, and even show regression of preexisting diseases. As they adopt a modern diet, their disease risks escalate and their health deteriorates to that of the typical American within one to two generations. The further away from the original diet, the greater the likelihood of developing diseases of civilization. The longer people live on the modern diet, the earlier they show signs of degenerative diseases and the earlier they need to be screened for disease, such as diabetes, heart disease, and hypertension.

People who have adopted the Origin Diet in this book are proof that it's never too late to reap the benefits of your heritage. They lose weight, their blood cholesterol levels drop, their energy improves, they even sleep better and can reduce the amount of their medications (under the supervision of a physician, of course). It's obvious that avoiding disease and managing your waistline result from eating closer to your evolutionary roots!

Our genes—the blueprint within each cell that controls the body, mind, and emotions—are almost identical to the genes of our earliest ancestors who lived 40,000 or more years ago. Provide those genes with the right amount and types of nutrients and they function in tip-top shape, stacking the evolutionary deck in our favor for living healthily and robustly well past one hundred years. Supply those genes with the wrong compounds in the wrong amounts or combinations and the system breaks down, just as a car backfires, pings, and stalls when fed dirty gas.

The Five Stone Age Secrets

More than 99 percent of our genetic heritage is identical to that of our prehuman ancestors. Ninety-nine percent of the remaining 1 percent is identical to our ancient ancestors' prior to agriculture. Genetically speaking, our bodies need the same amount of nutrients that were needed by our Paleolithic ancestors. Our bodies thrive on the foods on which they evolved. Given an alien diet of only highly processed, calorie-packed foods, our wild bodies weaken, become diseased, age rapidly, and die. Just as we have not developed a defense against the blindness that results from a vitamin A deficiency or the scurvy resulting from too little vitamin C, we also have not yet evolved a defense against the excessive saturated fats, sugars, salt, and refined products and the lack of essential nutrients, fiber, and other health-enhancing compounds in whole foods in our current diets. Chronic disease, obesity, depression, mental decline, and low energy are only a few of the consequences of eating out of sync with our origins.

So what can you do? Basically, you have two choices:

1. Do nothing. Allow natural selection to work its magic. In other words, avoid exercise and keep eating a highly processed diet loaded with saturated fat. You can't drastically change an individual, only a species, so this option will take some time. Over the course of tens of thousands of years our descendants who thrive on tamed and processed diets might evolve into a new species that requires only fabricated, high-fat foods and sitting in recliner chairs. No telling what that species will look like, but one possibility is that far-future generations will be fat, soft, and less vigorous than our ancient ancestors.

2. Take control. We can incorporate the best of our origins with the most up-to-date knowledge of nutrition and health. This combination of Stone Age and "New" Age should give our bodies, minds, and spirits everything needed to maximize our health potentials.

We can't change our genes (at least not overnight) and no one wants to return to the club and the cave, but we can recapture what we've lost and reconnect with our natural balance by gleaning the best from both our inheritance and our modern lifestyle. All we must do is make a few simple changes in what we eat, how much we move, and how we live.

Our ancestors lived by a set of unspoken rules, so innate to their well-being that they were as natural as breathing. These rules can be distilled into the Five Stone Age Secrets:

STONE AGE SECRET #1

STAY STRONG AND LEAN. Our ancestors, including our most recent ancient grandparents who lived in the Paleolithic period just before agriculture, were as physically fit as today's athletes. They combined walking and running with activity similar to weight lifting and stretching. This active lifestyle is one reason why those who lived beyond their eighties remained robust, active, relatively disease free, and youthful. (How to put this secret into practice will be discussed in chapters 2, 4, and 6.)

STONE AGE SECRET #2

FOCUS ON WILD (NATURAL) FOODS. Up to 65 percent of our original diets were fresh fruits and vegetables, nuts, seeds, and other plants. Our ancient ancestors ate pounds of produce every day. The other 35 percent came from wild game, low in saturated fats and rich in polyunsaturated fats called the omega-3 fatty acids. Hundreds of studies spanning decades of research show that diets based on these foods are also the ones that lower disease risk, prevent obesity, boost energy and mood, improve mental function, and slow aging. (How to put this secret into practice is discussed in chapters 2 and 5.)

STONE AGE SECRET #3

STAY HEALTHY AND ALERT. The rules were clear for our ancient ancestors: stay healthy and pay attention or die. Those who failed to pay attention to ever-changing food supplies were at high risk of starvation. Those who failed to stay healthy became prey. Those who paid attention and stayed healthy lived to tell the tale and pass on their wisdom. Today, people who have rich vocabularies, nurture creative thinking, hunger for knowledge, and explore life by learning new skills keep their minds active. They also are less likely to develop Alzheimer's disease. People who take care of their bodies by eating well and exercising regularly have the best chances of living long and healthy lives. In short, our minds and bodies were meant to stay active at every age. (How to put this secret into practice is discussed in chapter 3.)

STONE AGE SECRET #4

HANDLE STRESS QUICKLY, THEN RELAX. Like our ancient ancestors, people living in modern-day hunter-gatherer societies work hard and play well. They balance days of intense physical activity with days of hanging around camp, relaxing, and resting. The modern rat race often leaves little room for this reflective time, but the natural rhythm of our bodies, still needing the inner peace that comes from rest, is upset when one stress is piled on top of another. A weekly time-out from this frantic pace is essential if we want to live in harmony with our heritage. (How to put this secret into practice is discussed in chapter 7.)

STONE AGE SECRET #5

BELONG TO A SUPPORTIVE TRIBE OF FAMILY AND FRIENDS. We are social animals, with a long heritage of communication, cooperation, and cohabitation. We survived and evolved giving and receiving love, being needed by others, contributing to the tribe. That connectedness is what gives life meaning and purpose, which probably explains why happily married people live longer than single people, or why people with strong social support have low risks of developing heart disease and high blood pressure, recover quickly from illness, adapt better to life's changes, and live the healthiest lives. (How to put this secret into practice is discussed in chapter 7.)

Back to the Future

We are not the icing on the evolutionary cake, just one more layer. The dietary and lifestyle choices we make today are one more link in the endless chain of evolution. Those of our descendants living in the year 10,000 will be those who are best adapted to cope with their new environment. We can pass on a legacy of health, vitality, and vigorous living, or we can undermine our children's hopes of survival. Eating and living well is a contribution to both our own lives and the lives of generations to come. Besides, as Patricia, who adopted the Origin Diet in this book, said, "It feels good to take good care of myself."

How Nutritionally Aligned Are You with Your Origins?

You can't start on a journey, no matter how good the map, until you know your place of origin. That's why it's important to take stock of your eating, exercise, and general living habits before making any changes to align yourself with your heritage. Once you have accurately assessed your current habits, you'll have a much clearer idea of how to incorporate the Origin Diet and other tips in this book into your life.

The following checklist provides a gauge of what habits need changing and what habits are already in tune with your origins. Answer each question by giving yourself a score between 0 and 2 (0 = never, 2 = always). To monitor your progress, recheck yourself periodically after you've adopted the Original Dozen of the Origin program.

GOOD HEALTH   **Your Score**

1. I am in excellent health.
2. I maintain a desirable weight.
3. I maintain a desirable percent body fat.
4. When I notice my weight creeping up more than about five pounds, I quickly jump into action, reducing my food intake and increasing my exercise.
5. I avoid tobacco and other people's smoke.
6. My total blood cholesterol is under 200 mg/d.

GOOD HEALTH   **Your Score**

  7. My blood pressure is normal.

  8. My blood sugar is normal.

EXERCISE

  9. I exercise at least five days a week for at least forty-five minutes each day.

10. I include at least three sessions a week of aerobic activity, such as walking, running, swimming, or bicycling, in my exercise program.

11. I include at least two sessions a week of strength training in my exercise program.

12. I include some stretching and flexibility exercises in my routine.

13. Besides exercise, I am physically active for at least 2 hours during the day (i.e., I take the stairs, park far from the store, garden on the weekends).

EATING HABITS

14. I average at least eight, preferably ten, daily servings of fruits and/or vegetables, not counting French fries or other fried potatoes (give yourself one point for every serving up to ten).

15. I eat whole grains, including whole grain breads, cereals, pastas, and crackers.

16. I average at least two servings daily of nonfat milk, milk products, and/or calcium-fortified soymilk/cheese.

17. My protein-rich foods are only poultry breast, fish, wild game, and/or legumes.

18. The fats in my diet come only from nuts, seeds, olive or canola oils, avocados, fish, olives, and/or nut butters.

EATING HABITS

19. My diet is high in fiber.
20. I eat mini-meals and snacks throughout the day so that no more than four hours go by between meals.
21. I avoid processed foods, sugary or fatty foods, refined grains, salty foods, or foods high in additives.
22. I drink at least eight glasses of water every day.
23. I use honey or maple syrup, not sugar, and only in moderation.
24. I avoid red meat, whole milk and fatty dairy products, butter, margarine, whipped toppings, and other sources of saturated fats.
25. I use fat-free alternatives to high-fat items, such as sour cream, mayonnaise, cream cheese, and salad dressing.
26. I bake, steam, broil, poach, or grill food, rather than fry, sauté, or use sauces and gravies that contain fat.
27. When I eat in restaurants, I order low-fat, healthy foods.
28. I bring nutritious foods with me when I'm away from home.
29. I drink alcohol in moderation or not at all.
30. I drink caffeinated coffee in moderation or not at all.
31. I add little salt in cooking or on my food.

SUPPLEMENTS

32. I take a moderate-dose multiple vitamin and mineral supplement every day.

SUPPLEMENTS   Your Score

33. On the days when I don't consume at least two calcium-rich foods, I take a calcium-magnesium supplement.
34. I take extra antioxidants, such as vitamin E or vitamin C supplements.
35. When I don't eat fish, I take fish oil supplements and add flaxseed meal to my diet.

REST AND RELAXATION

36. On the days when I don't exercise, I take that extra time to relax.
37. I spend quality time every day with family and/or friends.
38. I limit or avoid television.
39. I keep my mind active by trying new skills, taking classes, learning, or challenging myself.
40. I am important in others' lives.
41. The world is a better place because I'm in it.
42. I avoid stress when I can, quickly handle the stress I can't avoid, and use some form of stress-reduction when stress lingers.
43. I have a good sense of humor and laugh a lot.
44. I have a creative outlet, such as music, drawing, theater, writing in a journal.
45. I get outside to enjoy the fresh air.
46. I sleep well and wake rested.

YOUR TOTAL SCORE:

Your goal is to keep your score in the A range. Any statement with a score less than 2 is an area you might consider improving.

90 or more: You score an A. Congratulations. You're living in harmony with your heritage and should be rewarded with great health, lots of energy, a clear mind, low risk for most diseases, and longevity. Keep up the good work!

80 to 89: Good work. You scored a B. Pinpoint two or three areas where you could boost your score into the A range to improve your health.

70 to 79: You're passing with a C average, which means you have room for improvement. Set a goal to improve your score by 10 points within the next month.

60 to 69: With only a D average, you need to make some changes right away. Try to improve your score by 10 points each month for the next two months.

59 or less: You've failed the test. Time to start taking your health more seriously. Set a goal to gradually improve your score by 10 points every month for the next three months until you're eating, moving, and living more in tune with your evolutionary roots.

2

Our Original Diet

Imagine you are an invisible bystander at your Paleolithic grandparents' campsite. You've brought a backpack with you that contains your favorite familiar foods to sustain you on your journey. Much of what is going on around the campfire is familiar to you: people are grilling meat, steaming vegetables, sharing food with family and friends, and laughing, teasing, and talking. One group is singing. Children are pestering adults. The general commotion might remind you of a typical family get-together.

Yet you quickly become aware of how different what you've packed to eat is from what your ancient companions are eating. As you peel back the plastic foil on a granola bar, those around you are eating roasted roots gathered that morning. While you quench your thirst with a can of soda pop, these ancient people are drinking water brought back to camp from a nearby stream. You bite into a bologna sandwich on white bread with mayonnaise, while the smells of roasting meat wrapped in herbs fill the air. There's not a food box, wrapper, bottle, bag, tub, or jar in sight. Nor do you see a loaf of bread, a sugar bowl, a glass of milk, a stick of butter, or a potato chip. The only produce in your backpack is an apple, while those gathered around the campfire are feasting on bowls heaped with cooked leaves, tubers, stalks, nuts, and beans. You've brought cookies, a candy bar, and a doughnut to satisfy your sweet tooth, while fresh and dried fruits drizzled with a little honey are the only sweet treats for your Paleolithic friends.

For 99.9 percent of the time humans have lived on earth our diets comprised only wild game and plants. As a result, all of our pre-agriculture ancestors consumed fewer calories per mouthful, yet much more fiber, vitamins, minerals, and other health-enhancing compounds in foods called phytochemicals. Their diets were low in total and saturated fats and higher in special fats called omega-3 fatty acids, including arachidonic acid (AA), eicosapentaenoic acid (EPA), and docosahexaenoic acid (DHA). (I'll discuss these compounds in detail later in this chapter.)

These diets are more than just chance. As Michael Crawford, Ph.D., a physical anthropologist and director of Brain Chemistry and Human Nutrition at Hackney Hospital in London, says, "Nutrition is not just about good health . . . nutritional chemistry is a fundamental evolutionary force." With the exception of breathing, nothing has ever been or probably ever will be more important to our survival and evolution than food. To understand how our bodies work and how to keep them in top running order, we must understand the foods that fuel them best. Those foods are the ones on which our ancient ancestors evolved. They are quite different from our diets today.

How Do We Know What Our Ancestors Ate?

We can scarcely remember what we ate for breakfast yesterday, so how can we be so sure what our ancient ancestors ate hundreds of thousands of years ago? "There has been a lot of interest and research on the diets of our ancient ancestors, perhaps because identifying what hunter-gatherers ate tells us a lot about how they lived," says Lauri Hager, Ph.D., research affiliate at the Archeological Research Facility at the University of California, Berkeley. Granted, the evolutionary diet puzzle is far from complete, but anthropologists have pieced together a pretty clear picture of what our ancient ancestors probably ate based on: (1) archeological evidence; (2) studies of modern-day hunter-gatherer populations in Australia, Africa, and South America; and (3) the nutritional analysis of wild game and plants.

ARCHEOLOGICAL EVIDENCE

Since 1925, thousands of ancient human bone fragments, full skeletons, skulls, campsites, weapons, tools, burial graves, carved and engraved objects, musical instruments, paintings, and even footprints have been unearthed. More than two hundred fossil fragments, representing fifteen individuals, were found in one location alone. Dietary intakes can be inferred from these records by studying the following:

1. Dentition (the types of teeth and how they were worn down by chewing). For example, fossil records show that our ancient ancestors had a thin enamel coating on their teeth, which implies they ate varied diets of softer foods. There are none of the grit marks and heavy wear on the teeth associated with eating bark and tough fibrous plants found in other primates' diets.

2. Extensive evidence from around the world—but especially in Europe, Asia, Australia, Africa, and possibly the Americas—of tool making, including harpoons, hand axes, snares, fish hooks, and other weapons used to hunt, trap, and kill game and fish.

3. The animal bones found at ancient campsites. For example, animal bones with cut marks show that meat was removed from bones using the equivalent of knives. At another archeological site, scientists determined that a single carcass was shared among three different hearths hundreds of feet apart, suggesting a potluck not unlike our modern-day holiday feasts.

4. Fossilized pollen found near and at archeological sites, which provides invaluable evidence of the type of plants that grew and were eaten before and during the Paleolithic era.

Advances in technology allow scientists to accurately date archeological evidence and to trace genetic material (called mitochondrial DNA, or mtDNA) back hundreds of thousands of years. Researchers at the University of Virginia have analyzed hair samples for forms of carbon, nitrogen, sulfur, and other isotopes, which yield detailed information on people's diets dating back thousands of years. "From our analysis of the proteins in hair we've been able to identify that one group ate up to a third of its diet as plants, while up to 90 percent of another group's diet came from the sea," says Stephen Macko, Ph.D., professor of environmental science at the University of Virginia.

Scientists also can glean much about our ancestors' diets by where they placed their camps, since ancient sites are usually situated close to places where herds of wild game would have migrated or crossed streams. The evidence of hunting, ambushing of animals, cooking, and sharing of food is obvious from these sites, as well as from the ancient artwork left behind. There are remains of pits dug in the permafrost that served as natural freezers in which meat was stored; a detailed record of countless stone tools used to hunt game, fish, scrape meat from bones, and process food; and cave paintings that depict the hunt for wild game and even the gathering of honey.

MODERN HUNTER-GATHERERS

More than two hundred modern-day hunter-gatherer societies have been studied. These people range from the semidesert tribes, including the Alyawara and the Aborigines in Australia and the !Kung San of southern Africa, to the tropical forest dwellers such as Efe Pygmies in Zaire, the Agta of the Philippines, and the Ache in Paraguay; to the savanna grasslanders, including the Cuiva in Venezuela and the Hadza in East Africa.

The variety of foods these people consume, including wild game and uncultivated wild plants, is similar to the range of foods available to our ancient ancestors. Like our ancestors, men do much of the hunting and women do most of the gathering. Granted, these modern-day tribes are not perfect replicas of the past. Their lives and societies are much more complex and sophisticated than ancient tribes, yet they live without technology and offer close reflections of how people survived eons ago.

The world in which they live is not quite the same as that of our ancient ancestors who had free rein to choose the richest and most fertile locations to hunt, scavenge, and gather. Today's tribes are relegated to areas of the world—the deserts, the tropical forests, and the Arctic—that are undesirable to modern societies. Consequently, the diets of modern-day foragers are probably not as rich, plant life not as diverse, and game not as plentiful as our ancestors' diets.

Yet these people fare quite well. In fact, the claim that our ancient ancestors ate poorly and were at high risk of malnutrition is not supported by the evidence that many modern-day hunter-gatherers are healthy and eat varied, nourishing diets. For example, the !Kung San of Botswana live in a semiarid region of the Kalahari Desert in Africa, which experiences a drought every two to three years. It's a marginal environment (which is why they have been left alone), yet these people collect all the food they need year-round by spending no more than about nineteen hours a week in food gathering—and with only meager tools such as digging sticks for roots, bows and arrows, long poles and hooks for catching burrowing animals, and rope snares. They select from more than 84 species of fruit, 30 species of roots and bulbs, and 144 species of animals (including lion, cheetah, jackal, fox, hyena, mongoose, badger, otter, squirrel, warthog, eland, kudu, python, and lizard) within a short distance of their camps. With such an assortment, they can choose only the tastiest and most easily collected food. Imagine how much richer the diets of ancient peoples would have been, living in the world's most fertile, pristine regions, untouched by modern societies.

Of course, there is no universal diet among hunter-gatherers, just as there are no two Americans who eat exactly the same. The 90-percent meat diet of the Eskimos is as different from the 90-percent plant diet of the Aborigines as a vegan diet is different from a fast-food diet. Yet, common patterns prevail when studying hunter-gatherer populations, which when pooled provide a composite diet not unlike how we have arrived at a typical American diet, which is an average of our society's eating habits.

In general, modern-day foragers consume between 20 and 35 percent of their diets as meat and the remaining 65 to 80 percent from plants.

This corresponds closely to the archeological data. "Fruits, roots, legumes, nuts, and other plants comprised about sixty-five to seventy percent of our ancient ancestors' diets, with very lean wild game and eggs making up the difference," says Dr. S. Boyd Eaton, "which is approximately the same ratio of animal to plants consumed by modern-day hunter-gatherers."

The old adage to eat a variety of foods finds its rationale in an eating style that dates back to the very origins of our species and is a basic tenet of all modern-day hunter-gatherer populations. For example, the Alyawara eat 102 different plant species (36 types of seeds, 32 types of flowers, 26 types of fruit, and 8 roots). The Tlokwa in Botswana eat 126 species of plants, including 22 leaves and stalks, 31 roots, 47 fruits, 23 barks and resins, and 3 types of mushrooms. The Ache select from more than 90 edible plants and animals. In industrialized societies today, eating a variety of foods is misconstrued to mean eating a wide range of refined and processed foods, when it really should mean eating a wide selection of unprocessed foods.

An even greater diversity of plants and animals was available to our ancient ancestors, and there is every reason to believe they took full advantage of the abundant food supply. Consider even the most recent accounts of buffalo in North America when settlers first began their migration westward. Buffalo herds were said to stretch from horizon to horizon and were so huge that it took days to pass by the entire herd. Scientists expect that our Paleolithic grandparents were such great hunters and feasted so regularly on mammoth that they drove the species to extinction about 12,000 years ago. North America once was home to camels, mammoth, great sloths, and horses, but all were hunted to extinction by Paleo-Indians long before Columbus ever set foot in the New World.

Finally, people living in modern-day hunter-gatherer societies provide us with a guesstimate of calorie intakes of our ancient ancestors. Based on the ratio of 35 percent animal and 65 percent plant foods and assuming a calorie density of about 112 calories/100 grams of plants and 129 calories/100 grams of animal, Dr. Eaton estimates that our ancient ancestors consumed on average about 3,000 calories daily. This fits into the framework of current primitive tribes, such as the Ache, who consume between 2,600 and 5,400 calories a day.

THE NUTRITION CONTENT OF WILD GAME AND PLANTS

Nutritional analysis has been completed on more than eighty-five different wild game animals, including the wild boar, bison, eland, kangaroo, oryx, and deer, and more than six hundred species of wild plants consumed by modern hunter-gatherer populations. This data, combined with extensive information on what hunter-gatherer populations eat and the ever-expanding archeological record, allow us to paint a lively, detailed picture of what our ancient ancestors ate, as well as compare that original diet to our current eating habits.

The Original Dozen: Living in Balance with Our Evolutionary Roots

A wealth of evidence, both direct and indirect, now exists on the types and amounts of foods on which our bodies evolved and thrive. We also have solid information on the types of lifestyles, activity levels, and social customs we need to feel comfortably "at home" and fully human, alive, well, and vigorous. Modern-day hunter-gatherers who live within this evolutionary balance, as well as our most ancient ancestors, live essentially free from chronic disease, maintain ideal body weights throughout life, live robustly into old age, have little or no incidence of emotional problems such as depression or anxiety, and show little loss of memory and thinking ability as they age. As tribal people adopt westernized lifestyles, their risk of diabetes, high blood pressure, heart disease, cancer, obesity, depression, even suicide escalates. If they return to tribal habits, their disease risk decreases.

The good news is that even though we've drifted far from our evolutionary roots, we can swing the pendulum back to a healthier way of life without too much effort. Basically, the guidelines are easy and are

THE ORIGINAL DOZEN

Do you want to fine-tune your life so it's more in balance with your evolutionary roots? Here are the twelve steps back to your future.

1. Consume eight to ten servings of a variety of rainbow-colored fruits and vegetables every day, or at least two at every meal and snack.

2. Carbohydrates are the mainstay of the diet and come from a variety of starchy vegetables, whole grains, fruits, legumes, and honey. Your fiber intake should average about 50 grams or more a day.

3. To cut back on saturated fat and boost your ratio of unsaturated to saturated fats, consume only skinless poultry breast, fish, shellfish, and wild game as sources of meat in the diet. Choose only fat-free milk products.

4. Healthful dietary fats come from the omega-3 fatty acids in fish, wild game, walnuts, and flaxseed meal and the unsaturated fats in nuts, avocados, olives, and olive and canola oils.

5. Graze, don't gorge, consuming five to six mini-meals over the course of the day.

6. Avoid or limit processed foods that include too much sugar, refined flours, salt, and additives.

7. Drink water, at least eight glasses a day.

8. If your weight creeps up by five pounds or more, voluntarily do what your ancestors were forced to do—create a temporary food shortage by lowering calorie intake and increasing daily activity.

9. Supplement responsibly.

10. Exercise vigorously five days a week and balance activity with days of rest.

11. Set aside time every week to spend with friends and family.

12. Avoid unnecessary stress and effectively handle the stress you can't avoid.

outlined in the Original Dozen (see box on page 38). Here's a detailed explanation of why the steps pertaining to diet (steps 1 through 9) are the steps that bring balance back to your health, energy level, weight, and life.

Four Pounds of Produce

Imagine a banquet table heaving under the weight of cooked wild game and an abundance of vegetables. There are bowls of leaves, fruits, nuts, beans, and roots. Baskets of tubers, stalks, bulbs, berries, melons, and flowers. You also see platters of cooked fungi, seaweed, clover root, salmonberries and their greens, and wild grasses, such as wild wheat and wild rice. There are even edible plants you don't recognize, such as the inner bark of cottonwood, thimbleberry shoots, fireweed, wood fern root, lupine root, bracken, and lamb's-quarters.

Our ancient ancestors thrived on an abundance of fresh plants, untouched by pesticides or additives. "Our Paleolithic ancestors consumed three or more times the amount of plant foods that we do," says Dr. Eaton. That means ten servings or more daily, or the equivalent of three to four pounds of produce. But, according to Susan Krebs-Smith, Ph.D., research nutritionist at the National Cancer Institute in Bethesda, Maryland, most people eat fewer than five servings daily. The top-ranking vegetable, averaging more than one serving daily is—you guessed it—potatoes, which are eaten fried approximately half the time. Nutrient-rich dark green leafy vegetables eaten by the pounds by our ancient ancestors make it to the twenty-first-century plate less than twice a week.

VITAMIN AND MINERAL GOLD MINES

Fruits and vegetables are the most nutrient-dense foods in the diet, so it's no wonder our bodies evolved on diets containing three times more vitamin B_2, two times more folic acid, eight times more vitamin C (up to 600 milligrams daily), and twice as much (about 10,000 IU) of beta carotene daily compared to modern diets. The abundance of dark green leafy vegetables in our ancestors' diets also accounts for their high calcium intake, estimated at about 1,900 milligrams daily, according to Dr. Eaton. Wild plants are also high in magnesium, iron, zinc, manganese, and vitamin B_1. Even wild grass seeds contain 50 percent more protein than domesticated wheat. Modern-day foragers who eat similar levels of plants also consume diets rich in vitamins and minerals. The fact that our bodies have thrived on pounds of nutrient-packed produce for hundreds of thousands of years explains why plant-derived nutrients, such as beta carotene, vitamin C, vitamin E, and the B vitamins, are nontoxic even at high doses, while some nutrients typically consumed in meat and milk, such as vitamin A (in liver) and vitamin D (in fortified milk), can accumulate to toxic levels when consumed in excess.

Much of the produce was eaten within hours of foraging and with little or no processing, which would maximize its nutritional content and would have produced a super-strong defense system against just about every form of degenerative disease. Today, these levels of vitamins and minerals are likely only if people take supplements.

PHYTOCHEMICAL POWERHOUSES

The phytochemical levels of our ancient ancestors' diets would have been off the charts by today's standards. Phytochemicals are health-enhancing compounds other than vitamins and minerals that prevent cancer, possibly boost the immune system, and protect against aging and heart disease. They're found only in unprocessed, natural foods—from fruits, vegetables, garlic, and soybeans to walnuts, wheat germ, and green tea. "Phytochemicals have completely changed the way we view foods. It's no longer appropriate to evaluate a food solely on its vitamin, mineral, and fiber content," says Mark Messina, Ph.D., associate professor at Loma Linda University.

Preliminary evidence already shows, for example, that a phytochemical called gingerol in ginger is a potent antioxidant, that the lignans in whole grains enhance fiber's protective effects against colon cancer, and that phenolic compounds in green tea might be major players in pro-

How Our Current Nutrient Intakes
Compare to Our Ancestors'

Our bodies evolved on levels of vitamins and minerals that are difficult to get today from diet alone. Dr. S. Boyd Eaton at Emory University in Atlanta has estimated our ancestors' intakes based on diets of 35 percent lean wild meat and 65 percent wild plants. Here's how they compare to modern nutrient recommendations and current intakes.

VITAMINS	OUR EVOLUTIONARY DIETS	RDA*	CURRENT INTAKES*
Vitamin A (RE—retinal equivalent)	17.2	4.8–6.0	7.02–8.48
Beta carotene (mg)	5.56	———	2.00–2.57
Vitamin E (mg)	32.8	8–10	7–10
Vitamin B_1 (mg)	3.91	1.1–1.5	1.08–1.75
Vitamin B_2 (mg)	6.49	1.3–1.7	1.34–2.08
Folic acid (mcg)	357	400	149–205
Vitamin C (mg)	604	60	77–109

MINERALS			
Calcium (mg)	1,956	800–1,200	500–720
Iron (mg)	87.4	10–15	9–11
Potassium (mg)	10,500	3,500	2,500
Sodium (mg)	768	500–2,000	4,000–20,000
Zinc (mg)	43.4	12–15	10–15
Fiber (g)	100–150	20–35	10–20

*Food and Nutrition Board, National Research Council: *Recommended Dietary Allowances,* tenth edition 1989, eleventh edition 1999.

tecting against heart disease. Other phytochemicals include the polyphenols like camosol in rosemary leaves or curcumin in mustard and curry, the flavonoids like quercetin in berries and onions, or rutin in citrus fruits, and kaempferal in kale and other greens. These and 12,000 other phytochemicals work as teams with nutrients and fiber to strengthen the body's defenses against disease.

Since our bodies evolved on diets that contained pounds, not ounces, of produce, it's likely our bodies function best on a high level of these phytochemicals. "The Dietary Guidelines suggest up to five servings of vegetables and four servings of fruit daily; that's nine servings a day from a very conservative recommendation," says Jeffrey Blumberg, Ph.D., professor of nutrition at the USDA Human Nutrition Research Center on Aging at Tufts University in Boston. But what is an optimal intake? According to Winston Craig, Ph.D., R.D., chairman and professor of nutrition at Andrews University in Michigan, "We don't know what an optimal dose is when it comes to phytochemicals, but we do know that the more phytochemical-rich fruits, vegetables, and whole grains you eat, the more protection you get." Based on the ancient diets on which we evolved, most of us should triple our current intakes to approach the level needed to sustain optimal health.

FIBER FITNESS

With our ancestors eating such a wide array of fruits, vegetables, legumes, nuts, and grasses, it's no wonder they consumed at least 100 grams of fiber every day. While this level might seem strange to us, accustomed to highly refined diets, in reality it is our current fiber intakes of 10 to 20 grams that are abnormal by evolutionary standards. The types of fiber in ancient diets also differ from current fiber intakes, since the fiber in fruits, vegetables, and legumes is higher in soluble fibers, such as pectin, hemicellulose, and gums. These fibers curb blood sugar and cholesterol levels and normalize intestinal bacteria.

QUALITY CARBS

Starchy vegetables, such as roots and tubers, fruits, and legumes, provided the main source of calories—carbohydrates—in our evolutionary diets. Carbohydrates in primitive tribal diets even today average about 50 percent of total calories, which is similar to current Western recommendations. However, all the carbohydrates on which our bodies

The Top 20 Plus Phytochemicals:
Why You Need Them and Where You'll Find Them

FOOD	PHYTOCHEMICAL	FUNCTION
Fruit	Ferulic acid	Decreases nitrosamines
	Caffeic acid	Solubilizes carcinogens
Dark green/ orange vegetables	Carotenoids: lutein, lycopene, alpha or beta carotene, canthaxanthin	Antioxidants
Berries/nuts/ grapes	Ellagic acid	Antioxidant; stops DNA mutations
Green tea	Flavonoids	Antioxidants
Cruciferous vegetables	Indoles	Modulate estrogen, decrease cancer risk
	PIETC	Inhibits lung cancer
	Phenols: flavonoids	Antioxidants
	Sulforaphane	Inhibits cancer growth
Citrus	Monoterpenes: esp. limonene	Inhibit mammary cancer
Tomatoes/ green peppers/ strawberries	P-Coumaric acid, Chlorogenic acid, Lycopene	Inhibits carcinogens, decreases nitrosamines Protects DNA (antioxidant)
Beans/soy	Saponins	Decrease cholesterol
	Phytosterols	Slow colon cancer growth
	Phytoestrogens	Alter estrogen, decrease breast cancer
Garlic/onions	Sulfur compounds	Inhibit cancer, decrease heart disease, stimulate immunity
Wild purslane	Phosphatidylserine	Boosts memory, thinking

evolved came from unprocessed, high-fiber, nutrient-packed wild plants. In contrast, our food supply has lurched and crept in a constant direction toward energy-packed, increasingly nutrient-poor processed grains, sugar, and fried starchy vegetables, so that today carbohydrate is synonymous with sweets, white bread, egg noodles, and French fries. "The emphasis today is on grains, when in fact grains were a small part of the diets of humans for 99 percent of their evolutionary history," says Dr. Lauri Hager.

Compared to whole grains, which are the closest foods we have to wild grass seeds, processed carbohydrates supply no fiber, are much lower in nutrients, and often pack a much higher calorie punch. As you'll see in chapter 3, these processed starches also aggravate diabetes and other degenerative diseases, while wild foods lower our risk for most diseases.

The Bison Burger

Although plants were the dietary mainstay, our ancestors also ate their fair share of meat. They hunted, trapped, and ambushed anything that moved. They planned their hunts in advance, knew annual migratory patterns and cycles, coordinated their hunting efforts, waited in blinds and near water holes, and even scavenged meat when there was none to kill. They feasted on reindeer, shrew, mammoth, wild cattle, antelope, oxen, horse, fox, beaver, rabbit, ibex, red deer, caribou, bison, boar, fish, shellfish, sea mammals, and birds (duck, pigeon, and grouse, to name a few). In South America, they ate llamas, horses, giant sloths, and rheas (birds that resemble small ostriches). Along the coast of southern Africa, they hunted antelope, giant buffalo, eland, wildebeest, and hartebeest. In Australia, they ate emus, wallabies, kangaroo, and a variety of now-extinct megamarsupials. Then they probably sat around the campfire in the evening and told overblown stories of the danger and daring of the kill.

But unlike today's meat that comes from domesticated animals and is high in saturated fat, the meat on ancient plates was only wild game, which is low in fat (4 percent fat versus 25 to 30 percent in domesticated meat), very low in saturated fat, has five times more polyunsaturated fat, a high concentration of omega-3 fatty acids, and fewer calories than most meat today. Wild game also supplies more protein per ounce than do domesticated meats.

Meat is an ideal food for our species. Packed with calories, B vitamins, trace minerals, and protein, it is the densest source of nutrition in our diets. Whether our ancestors lived on the savanna or in the Arctic, in the rain forest or along the coast, wild game was plentiful and provided the most nutrition for the least effort. Because a large carcass can feed an entire tribe, meat was the ideal food for sharing with friends and family, for courting the ladies, tending the sick, and gaining power within the community (the best hunter often is the most honored and revered). Meat was as much political as it was nutritional.

GOOD FATS/BAD FATS

Wild game gives a whole new meaning to the term "animal fats." Considered the bane of our dietary existence today and linked to disease such as heart disease and cancer, meat has received a lot of bad press. But the meat on which our bodies envolved was very different from the meat available in grocery stores today. It supplied our ancestors with an entirely different array of calorie-rich fats essential not only to survival of one generation, but to the evolution of our entire species. The fact that the human body absorbs 95 percent of the dietary fat consumed is evidence that this concentrated source of calories was hard to come by in Paleolithic times.

The fat in and around the muscle of wild game constitutes no more than 2 percent of muscle weight and contains two times more polyunsaturated fat than saturated fat; thus, its fat composition resembles nuts more than beef. In contrast, a typical cut of pork today contains up to 30 percent fat by weight, more than three quarters of its calories come from fat, and more than twice as much of that fat is saturated than polyunsaturated fat. Take, for example,

- lamb, which has eight times more fat than does wild goat;
- pork loin, which has ten times the fat of buffalo;
- ham, which has more than 18 times more fat than gazelle;
- even chicken, which has ballooned from only 2.4 percent fat at the turn of the twentieth century to 22 percent fat by weight and up to 84 percent fat calories today. A far cry from wild partridge, which is 36 percent fat calories!

Wild game is also unique in that it contains up to 2.7 percent of its fat as omega-3 fatty acids, a type of polyunsaturated fat that lowers disease risk. Domesticated meat has no omega-3 fatty acids. How could meat be so nutritionally different? The difference comes from what the animals eat. Just as the composition of mother's milk and our own body fat is a direct reflection of the fats we consume in our diets, so animal tissue also mirrors dietary intake. Wild animals feast on wild seeds, acorns, nuts, leaves, and woody material rich in omega-3 fatty acids, while domesticated animals feed on grasses and grains devoid of these important fats.

For our ancestors, the high intake of omega-3-rich plants and game provided a ratio of plant oils called omega-6 fatty acids (from seeds and nuts) to omega-3 fatty acids of somewhere between 4:1 to 1:1. Today, we eat lots of foods processed in omega-6-rich vegetable oils, such as safflower, soybean, and corn oil. We smear margarine on our toast, use shortening in baking, and swing into drive-through windows for a quick lunch of fried foods. But we include very little omega-3-rich fish and no wild game in our daily diets. Consequently, we consume eleven times more omega-6-rich oils than we do omega-3 fats. Not to mention saturated fat, which is at levels never before consumed in the entire history of our species. As you'll read in chapter 3, this imbalance in our dietary fats is linked to increased rates of heart disease, cancer, depression, attention deficit disorder (ADD), osteoporosis, and even suicide.

Many scientists believe that if the diets of our ancient ancestors had been low in omega-3 fatty acids, we never would have developed our

A Meaty Matter

Wild game is as different nutritionally from domesticated meat as doughnuts are from whole grains.

ANIMAL	% POLYUNSATURATED FAT	% SATURATED FAT
Wild		
Eland	35	65
Giraffe	39	61
Grouse	60	40
Antelope	85	15
Bison	62	38
Deer	58	42
Boar	63	37
Domesticated		
Beef	2	98
Chicken	17	83
Pork	8	92

unique, complex nervous system, regardless of other social factors influencing our development. Our ancestors' brains increased threefold when consumption of omega-3-rich foods increased hundreds of thousands of years ago. These fats make up the majority of polyunsaturated fats in our brains, providing the structural components necessary for nerve and brain tissue to develop. Sixty percent of the structural material in our brains is fat, and 90 percent of the polyunsaturated fats are omega-3 fatty acids. To allow for the rapid increase in brain size that occurred hundreds of thousands of years ago, our ancestors had to have ample access to the omega-3 fatty acids, including DHA and EPA. Culture, speech, and tool use developed as a result of our expanding brains.

Today, we know that the brains and eyes of infants fed diets low in omega-3s do not develop properly. In addition, human brain size was 11 percent greater ten thousand years ago before the discovery of agriculture, which caused a dramatic drop in our intakes of omega-3 fatty

The Omega-3s and Our Brains

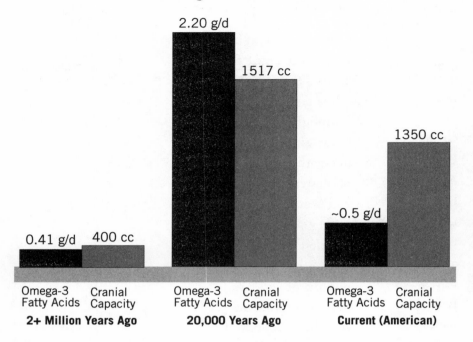

Human brain size parallels our consumption of omega-3 fatty acids, and was 11% greater when we consumed a hunter-gatherer diet of wild game and plants.

acids. Our ancient ancestors consumed about 12.6 grams of omega-3s every day; according to the U.S. Department of Agriculture, most people currently consume only 0.5 to 1.4 grams daily. "We are consuming a significantly lower amount of fatty acids than the recommendations made by international agencies," says Penny Kris-Etherton, Ph.D., R.D., distinguished professor of nutrition at Pennsylvania State University. "Recommendations to achieve the proposed EPA and DHA intake will require a two- to threefold increase in omega-3-rich foods, such as fish," adds Dr. Kris-Etherton. While matching our ancient ancestors' intake for these oils would be difficult, research shows that including even a few servings a week of omega-3-rich fish can reduce disease risk and improve mood. (See chapter 3 for more information on how the omega-3 fatty acids affect our mental, emotional, and physical health and chapter 5 for ways to increase your intake of omega-3s.)

CHOLESTEROL

Wild game might be low in fat and saturated fat, but it contains about the same amount of cholesterol found in domesticated animals. It's likely that our ancestors consumed as much as 500 milligrams of cholesterol a day, which is far above the current recommendation to limit cholesterol to 300 milligrams or less. Despite this high intake, there is no evidence that our ancient ancestors suffered from heart disease. Modern-day hunter-gatherers also often consume similar intakes, yet maintain blood cholesterol levels under 150 mg/dl, which is well below the American average of 205 mg/dl, and they show no signs of heart disease.

While dietary cholesterol has been linked to an increased risk of developing heart disease, it is likely that it is not so much the cholesterol as it is the high amount of saturated fat in the same foods. In fact, all foods high in cholesterol—from meat to dairy products—are also high in saturated fat, with the exception of eggs, which are high in cholesterol but low in saturated fat. Modern-day hunter-gatherers and our ancient grandparents might have eaten their fair share of cholesterol, but they ate very little saturated fat and an abundance of heart-protective foods, such as high-fiber fruits, vegetables, legumes, and wild grains. They also were very physically active, which extensive research shows lowers body weight and disease risk.

Recent research from Harvard Medical School found that nondiabetics who followed a low-fat diet could consume up to an egg a day with no apparent harm to their hearts. Since a single egg contains approximately 270 milligrams of cholesterol, a varied diet that regularly included eggs would easily bring the total day's cholesterol intake to 400 to 500 milligrams, well within our ancestors' intakes.

TFA-FREE

Never did a processed fat grace our ancestors' lips until the twentieth century, when food manufacturers began hydrogenating vegetable oils. Margarine and shortening are liquid vegetable oils made creamy when manufacturers convert some of the unsaturated fats into saturated ones. To do this, hydrogens are added to the long strings of carbon atoms that compose the fat molecule, hence the terms "hydrogenation" and "hydrogenated vegetable oils."

Hydrogenation does more than just add a few hydrogens here and there; it changes the structure of the polyunsaturated fats, converting them from their natural "cis" shape (like a U) to an abnormal "trans" shape (like a Z). Only traces of these unnatural trans fatty acids (TFAs) were in our diets up until the twentieth century. Now we consume 10 to 20 grams of TFAs a day. Daily intakes of up to 100 grams are possible if a person regularly eats potato chips, cookies, crackers, or fried fast foods. Yet our bodies have not had time to evolve a defense against them; consequently, consuming TFAs is linked to numerous health problems, from heart disease and suppressed immunity to infertility and diabetes. (Read more about TFAs in chapter 3.)

THE ISSUE OF PROTEIN

Current nutrition advice tells us to limit protein to 12 to 15 percent of total calories or about 0.75 grams of protein for every 2.2 pounds of body weight (i.e., 51 grams for a 150-pound person). Our ancient ancestors ate much more than that, or up to 30 percent of calories from protein (approximately 2.0 to 3.0 grams of protein for every 2.2 pounds of body weight or 136 to 204 grams for a 150-pound person). However, this is one ancient dietary habit that might not transfer to our modern-day lives.

Our ancestors maintained significantly greater muscle mass than humans today, muscle mass comparable to professional athletes. Protein-rich diets would help build and maintain this muscle, while even a very fit nonathlete today has no need for that level of protein. Today, westernized people who consume high-protein diets do not build more muscle, they merely excrete more protein by-products, such as urea, in their urine, which increases their risk for kidney stones. In addition, high-protein diets increase urinary loss of calcium, increasing a person's risk for developing osteoporosis. While not a problem in the Paleolithic diet that contained as much as 1,900 milligrams of calcium each day, our high-protein, low-calcium diets today present a problem for bone health.

In short, our modern-day bodies evolved on protein-rich diets, but unless we maintain the level of intense physical exertion necessary to warrant that protein intake, eating more than 20 percent of calories from protein presents more of a health risk than a benefit.

The Original Low-Salt Diet

Then there's salt (sodium chloride). Our ancestors averaged only 770 milligrams of sodium each day, but up to 10,500 milligrams of potassium (a sodium to potassium ratio of 1:13). Today, we've reversed the ratio, consuming much more sodium and a lot less potassium. We average 2,300 to 6,900 milligrams of sodium daily, and some people nibble on enough salty processed foods to boost sodium intake above 20,000 milligrams a day. We are the only nonmarine animal to eat diets so high in salt. Primitive cultures today, where people consume diets similar to our ancient ancestors' with ten times the potassium to sodium, have low blood pressure rates, almost no incidence of hypertension, and their blood pressures don't rise with age as ours do.

While the heavy-handed salt shaker at home contributes to our salty diets, by far the bulk of our salty intake, or approximately 75 percent, is added for us by industry in processed foods. Only 10 percent of the salt we consume occurs naturally in food. For example:

- An ear of corn naturally has 3 milligrams of sodium; compare that to the 214 milligrams in a small bag of corn chips or the 255 milligrams in a bowl of corn flakes.
- A baked potato supplies only 6.8 milligrams of sodium compared to 506 milligrams in an equal weight of potato chips or 373 milligrams in the same amount of packaged potatoes au gratin.

- Or take oatmeal, which supplies less than 1 milligram of sodium compared to 250 milligrams in a granola bar and 458 milligrams in an oatmeal cookie.
- Even vegetables become salt mines when processed. While raw broccoli supplies 23 milligrams of sodium in a three-ounce serving, the same portion of packaged broccoli with cheese sauce packs in 134 milligrams of sodium, while an equal serving of cream of broccoli soup supplies 280 milligrams.

In general, the more a food is processed, the higher its salt, sugar, and/or fat content and the further it is from our original diet's nutritional content.

Is It Worth Its Weight in Salt?

Five to 6 grams of salt (or 2,400 milligrams of sodium), the equivalent of a teaspoon, is currently considered the maximum recommended daily intake, while our ancestors thrived on intakes one third of this amount. A diet high in processed foods would easily exceed this limit several times!

FOOD	SODIUM (MG)
Tomato sauce, canned (1 cup)	1,480
Ham and Swiss sandwich (5 ounces)	1,350
Spaghetti sauce, bottled (1 cup)	1,200
Potatoes au gratin (1 cup)	1,065
Soy sauce (1 tablespoon)	1,030
Pinto beans, canned (1 cup)	1,000
Turkey pot pie, frozen (8 ounces)	1,000
Macaroni and cheese, frozen (8 ounces)	970
Fast food hamburger	900
Chicken soup, canned (1 cup)	870
Imitation crabmeat (3 ounces)	715
Canadian bacon (1½ ounces)	700

Sweet Origins

Our bodies evolved on small amounts of carbohydrate-rich sweets, mostly honey and fruits. But these were seasonal and scarce: so scarce, in fact, that cave paintings show our ancient ancestors risking the vengeance of the hive and exerting considerable effort just to steal a lick of this sweet syrup. Even in modern-day hunter-gatherer tribes, honey is available only for a few months out of the year.

Today, each one of us eats more refined sugar in a day than our ancient ancestors ate in a lifetime. The latest statistics show we produce enough sugar in this country to feed every man, woman, and child 152 pounds of refined sweeteners every year, including table sugar, high fructose corn syrup, dextrose, and more. That's 25 pounds per person a year more than was produced in the 1980s. Not all of that sugar is actually eaten, but according to diet surveys, the average American consumes at least 20 teaspoons of refined sugar every day, or about 16 to 20 percent of total calories. That's at least 146,000 sugar calories a year, or the amount of energy needed to run more than a marathon every week all year-round.

Americans' fear of fat has been a boon to the sugar industry, as has our escalating sweet tooth. Fat-free desserts use extra sugar to make up for the flavor lost when fat is removed. But even nondesserts are sweet. Some fruited yogurts have the sugar equivalent of a candy bar, and cinnamon-apple instant oatmeal contains up to eight teaspoons of sugar per serving. Even a serving of canned franks and beans contains more than three teaspoons of sugar. Many processed foods, from salad dressing and cereals to bottled spaghetti sauce and crackers, contain added sugar.

Whether sugar directly causes disease or obesity is a controversial issue. However, one thing is not debatable: Every time you put a sugary food in your mouth, you're missing the opportunity to eat a food more in tune with your evolutionary roots. One study from Tulane University in New Orleans reported that children who ate lots of sugar consumed significantly lower amounts of protein, vitamins, and minerals. Another study from North Dakota State University found that as sugar consumption increases, intake of protein, B vitamins, iron, magnesium, and vitamins D and E decrease. Dr. Krebs-Smith and colleagues have noted that the latest U.S. Department of Agriculture Continuing Survey of Food Intakes by Individuals (CSFII) shows that a measly one out of every one hundred people meet even minimum standards for dietary adequacy. Yet obesity is on the rise, with the average American seven pounds heavier today than he or she was a decade ago. Consuming calorie-dense foods, such as sweets, is certainly a major contributor to malnutrition in the face of overnutrition.

Drinking from the River of Life

Our bodies are more water than anything else. In fact, 50 to 70 percent of us is water, depending on how much weight is fat and how much is muscle. More than 85 percent of our blood, 70 percent of our muscles, and 75 percent of our brains is water. Water surrounds and fills every cell in our bodies. Water acts as a solvent, coolant, lubricant, and transport agent. It's needed to regulate body temperature, remove waste products of metabolism and toxic compounds, carry nutrients, maintain blood and lymph volume, and provide the medium for all the body's billions of chemical reactions to occur. Water even helps fend off fatigue, keeps the skin moist, fills us up, and curbs hunger pangs, thus aiding in weight management. Patricia adopted the Origin Diet and commented, "Lots of time I found I was really thirsty when I thought I wanted to eat, so putting a jug of water close by is a great way to cut back on unwanted calories and food."

Every major system in our bodies begins to break down when water is in short supply. For example, if your muscles lose even 3 percent of their water, they lose 10 percent of their ability to contract and 8 percent of their speed. Concentration and reaction times drop; stamina and resistance to disease are also compromised. "Your body just won't work right without enough water. It can't rid itself of waste products, so toxins accumulate. The cells can't function properly when water balance is disrupted," warns Nancy Clark, M.S., R.D., nutrition coach at Sports-Medicine Brookline in Brookline, Massachusetts.

Our bodies need water more than anything except for oxygen. They evolved on an unlimited supply of it. All the water our bodies need must come from the foods we eat and the beverages we drink. Since we lose at least 2½ pints (5 cups) of water as urine every day, not to mention the amount lost in perspiration and respiration, we need to replace that by drinking the same amount or more of water every day. As long as a person is healthy, it's almost impossible to drink too much of this life-giving beverage.

Today, we're more concerned about watering our lawns than ourselves. Soft drinks are the beverage of choice, with consumption surpassing water, milk, coffee, tea, fruit juices, or any beverage. While our bodies evolved on water, the average man, woman, and child now pours more than fifty-two gallons of soft drinks into his or her body every year. "Children are consuming 8 percent of their calories from soft drinks, which is an enormous amount of wasted calories," warns William Dietz, M.D., Ph.D., director of nutrition and physical activity for the Centers for Disease Control and Prevention in Atlanta. Contributing nothing but calories, soft drinks either replace the nutrient-packed foods our bodies need or they are consumed in excess of our calorie needs, adding to the escalating rates of obesity. If they're caffeinated, soft drinks have a slightly dehydrating effect, further increasing our need for what we should have been drinking in the first place—water.

Those Little Vices:
Caffeine, Alcohol, and Tobacco

The legal drugs of choice in our culture—caffeine (in coffee, cola, and tea), alcohol, and nicotine in tobacco—probably played a minor role, if any, in our ancient ancestors' lives. "A small amount of alcohol probably snuck into our ancient grandparents' diets when fruit or honey spontaneously fermented," says Dr. Lauri Hager. Some ancient groups might even have made ceremonial beverages with these fermented juices. But widespread use of alcoholic beverages was not part of our heritage until after the development of agriculture. Modern-day hunter-gatherer populations only began drinking alcoholic beverages after being introduced to them by more advanced societies. If we evolved on small amounts of alcohol, this would fit recent findings that a few glasses of wine each week lower heart-disease risk, while two or more alcoholic beverages a day raise a woman's risk for breast cancer.

Caffeine in small doses is likely to have been part of our ancestors' diets, since it is available in a variety of plants around the world. "Cocoa beans have been found in Maya ruins, suggesting that these ancient peoples at least had chocolate," says Dr. Hager. Coffee, a primary source of caffeine in today's diets, was rare to nonexistent in pre-agriculture societies. In fact, coffee was first discovered only around 1,150 years ago, when an Arab goatherd in southern Ethiopia reportedly noticed that his goats were more frisky after chewing the beanlike seeds from a tropical shrub. Many teas contain caffeine, and it is likely that these brews graced the lips of more than one of our ancient grandparents.

Tobacco is entirely foreign to all species, including humans. While Aborigines chew tobacco, no other modern-day foragers use the uncultivated plant. Wild tobacco would have been available only seasonally in some regions of the world. Tobacco was first cultivated in the Americas about five thousand years ago, but Europeans, Africans, and Asians had no exposure to it until it was brought back by Columbus. Cigarettes were not manufactured until the late nineteenth century. With no evolutionary exposure to this leaf, it's no wonder that the consequences of using tobacco are so devastating to health and longevity.

Beyond the Dietary Guidelines

In the past several decades, national dietary recommendations have slowly progressed toward a style of eating that reflects the ones on which humans evolved. While in the 1970s the Basic Four Food Groups recommended we eat daily at least four fruits and vegetables, by the late 1980s, recommendations had increased that intake to a range of five to nine. Previous dietary recommendations emphasized grains, but more recent recommendations place more emphasis on whole grains. Hundreds of studies spanning decades of research show that diets resembling those on which we evolved—low in saturated fats and high in fiber-rich plant foods—lower our risk for developing heart disease, cancer, diabetes, hypertension, cataracts, and other physical problems; boost our moods; and help us live longer and healthier lives. "The gradual accumulation of damage to the body's tissues that we associate with aging and disease is often entirely preventable if people maintain a strong antioxidant defense. The first line of defense is to eat lots of fruits and vegetables," states Dr. Blumberg.

Yet our evolutionary diets were different from today's recommendations:

- They extend current diet advice by suggesting we eat not five to nine, but ten or more fresh fruits and vegetables.
- While current guidelines make no recommendations on the best produce, our evolutionary diet spells it out in no uncertain terms—choose the colorful produce, such as romaine lettuce, not iceberg; sweet potatoes, not French fries; and eat more broccoli, green peas, blueberries, strawberries, kiwi, and prunes. These are the selections that pack the greatest phytochemical and nutrient punch for the lowest calorie bang.
- We also thrive on whole grains, not refined grains, since our bodies evolved on fiber-rich wild grass seeds, not highly processed starch granules (see What Processing Has Done to Our Food on p. 58).
- Finally, the suggestion to eat a variety of foods means more than just snacking on a different convenience food every day. In fact, the word "processed" is not part of our heritage. Instead, we should choose a broad range of minimally processed, wholesome foods as often as possible, which automatically cuts back our intake of salt, sugar, calories, and fat.

Unlike current diet advice to consume two to three servings daily of lean meat, our bodies evolved on meat with a fat composition equivalent to that of nuts, salmon, seafood, and shellfish. Skinless poultry breast meat and wild game such as venison or elk also fit the low-saturated-fat requirements, as do legumes, such as cooked dried beans and peas, soy foods, and lentils. While current diet advice suggests limiting cholesterol, an evolutionary perspective shows that cholesterol is not a problem when saturated fat is very low, fiber-rich foods are the foundation of a healthy person's diet, and vigorous exercise is as natural as brushing your teeth.

WHAT PROCESSING HAS DONE TO OUR FOOD

Processing foods results in substantial losses of nutrients. For example:

- 48.9 percent of the vitamin B_6 is lost when seafood is processed.
- 77 percent of the vitamin B_6 is lost when vegetables are processed.
- Up to 78 percent of the pantothenic acid (a B vitamin) is lost when foods are processed.
- 86.5 percent of the vitamin E and 50 percent of the molybdenum are lost when wheat is refined.
- 81.7 percent of the manganese, 70.6 percent of the cobalt, and 40 percent of the zinc are lost when spinach is canned.
- 50 percent of the choline is lost when brown rice is refined.

DESIGNER, GENETICALLY ENGINEERED, AND FUNCTIONAL FOODS: CAVE DWELLER'S DREAM OR NIGHTMARE?

In an effort to boost the meager nutritional value of our overly processed foods, manufacturers are adding vitamins, minerals, herbs, and phytochemicals to new foods. These nutritionally fortified products are called functional foods, and they are likely to be the foods of the future, for better or for worse. Isolating specific health-enhancing compounds in whole foods, then transferring them to other foods, either by dumping them as additives into processed foods or by genetically altering whole-some foods, is the latest passion of researchers and industry. This is where the graying of the line between foods and medicine is most pronounced. It's also the most controversial trend.

In addition to the current concern that genetically engineered foods could harbor hidden allergens potentially deadly to highly allergic indi-viduals, there is also the issue of blindly messing with a good thing. "We know so little about optimal doses, interactions, or long-term conse-quences of most phytochemicals that to begin adding them haphazardly into pills or even concentrating them into other foods could produce any number of potentially toxic effects," warns Dr. Craig.

We've been consuming genetically engineered foods since 1994 in everything from tomatoes to baby foods and potato chips. Supplements, drinks, and energy bars are just the beginning of a wave of high-tech products packed with varying amounts of phytochemicals, probiotics, herbs, vitamins, and antioxidants. Watch this trend with a wary eye and don't be fooled by new products advertised as herb- or phytochemical-fortified mood enhancers, energy boosters, life extenders, or disease fighters. To eat in tune with your evolutionary roots, you're better off sticking with wholesome, unprocessed, real food, which is what your body craves anyway.

Stone Age Secrets #1 and #2: How to Stay Lean and Strong by Eating à la Natural

We can't return to the cave (nor would we want to!), mammoths and mastodon are extinct, and our fruits and vegetables are cultivated, not wild, yet we can still regain balance with our health and our food. For-tunately, our bodies are only concerned with getting the right amount of nutrients. The source is unimportant. Chicken breast is as good a source of low-fat protein as gazelle, salmon is as good a source of omega-3 fatty acids as eland, and you can get your vitamin C just as well from oranges as from wild greens.

The secret to regaining our evolutionary balance is to glean the best of our ancient ancestors' eating habits and combine those with the safe, abundant, nutritious foods available today. That means designing our diets based on a wide variety of fruits, vegetables, whole grains, legumes, nuts, seeds, fish, shellfish, poultry breast meat, and wild game when it's available. Cultivated produce contains lower levels of some minerals than do wild plants, so it is difficult to get the levels of calcium found in ancient times from plants alone. Since it is only the saturated fat in milk that is a health concern, there is good reason to include nonfat milk products in this eating plan, or to consume calcium- and vitamin-D-fortified soymilk.

As listed in the Original Dozen on page 38, minimize your intake of processed foods and you will automatically cut back on calories, fat, salt, and sugar and will find it much easier to attain and maintain a desirable weight. In addition, become a grazer like your ancient ancestors by evenly dividing those foods into mini-meals and snacks throughout the day, drink plenty of water, and put yourself on a temporary food shortage by lowering calories and increasing exercise when you see your weight creep up by a few pounds. As a result you will find, as everyone who has adopted this eating plan has found, that you have more energy and mental power, sleep better, suffer less from food cravings, and feel more vital. Chapter 5 will explain exactly how to put this evolutionary wisdom into modern-day practice.

3

Live Healthier, Live Longer

There is little room for argument with the proposal that health . . .
would be substantially improved by a diet and exercise schedule
more like that under which we humans evolved.

—JAMES V. NEEL, author of *Physician to the Gene Pool*

Every thirty-three seconds someone's loved one dies from heart disease.
It's the number-one cause of death in men and women, and risk escalates as we age. All of this suffering is rare to nonexistent in hunter-
gatherer populations, and there is no evidence that heart disease existed
in our pre-agricultural ancestors. Hunter-gatherers maintain blood cholesterol levels of 125 mg/dl, a level similar to that found in other primates, yet far below the average level of 205 mg/dl in our culture, where
one in every two people dies from heart disease. People who live and eat
in sync with evolutionary habits don't suffer from diabetes, stroke, hypertension, osteoporosis, obesity, and even cancer. Hearing loss, dental
caries, alcoholism, diverticulosis, and memory loss are also rare. People
who have adopted the Origin Diet in this book repeatedly comment
that it improves more than just disease risk.

Why Is This?

Are primitive people at low risk for chronic diseases because they just
don't live long enough? No. The signs of disease, such as elevated blood
glucose levels, fatty streaks in the arteries, and obesity, are present in our
youth. After age thirty-five, most people in Western cultures have the

beginnings of disease, including raised blood cholesterol and blood pressure, bone loss, and a gradual loss of immune function. These early symptoms aren't present in foragers. For example, although fatty streaks in the arteries are already present in teenagers in our culture, the same arteries in young hunter-gatherers are clear and supple. The initiation process of many diseases, such as atherosclerosis, where the artery walls are damaged and ripe for fatty deposits, is the same in all peoples. The difference is that the injury is quickly repaired in foragers, leaving no lasting damage, while it progresses in people living in Western cultures.

You also can't use the excuse that foragers have a genetic immunity to heart disease and other chronic disorders. When these people adopt Western habits, their body weight, blood cholesterol and blood pressure, and risk for heart disease, diabetes, hypertension, cancer, osteoporosis, and other degenerative diseases escalate. For example, when the Tarahumara Indians in Mexico, who have virtually no heart disease risk factors, consume Western-style diets, they have dramatic increases in blood cholesterol levels and body weights, which increase their risk for heart disease and other degenerative disorders. Disease risk drops when they return to their native lifestyles.

No Life of Riley

Granted, modern-day hunter-gatherers and our ancient foraging ancestors aren't examples of perfect health. Trauma was a major source of pain and disability. Infections, including respiratory, fungal, and parasitic infections, undermined health and caused death. Overexertion led to disability, just as it does today in people who don't take care of their bodies. Choosing to walk upright almost 4 million years ago, rather than on all fours like our ultra-ancient ancestors, brought with it backaches, knee problems, and even birthing complications (women's pelvises are narrower than other primates') that haunt us still.

But the health problems foragers face are ones Western societies can easily avoid or control through safety standards, sanitation, vaccinations, medical care, and preventive health care. What primitive people teach us is that the diseases that plague modern societies today are not inevitable. They're not even normal. They are exceptions to an evolutionary rule and red flags that show we have not adapted to our current lifestyles. The only adaptation to this lifestyle is chronic degenerative disease, and it can be avoided by embracing some of our past.

The same benefits are possible for anyone. Within just a few weeks of adopting the Origin Diet in this book, people lose weight, their cholesterol levels drop, energy levels improve, and cravings for sweets subside, and they sleep better and feel more mentally alert. "The best part was the results from my cholesterol test; I've never had results that low!" says Dolores. Some reduce medication dosages with the supervision of their physicians. "My general health improved and it's easier now to get out of bed in the morning and up from the table after meals, and even though I'm full, I don't have that tired feeling I used to have. I'm also sleeping better," says LeRoy. "My energy has been great ever since I switched to eating this way!" adds Tim.

In Our Own Defense: How Our Bodies Naturally Fight Disease and Aging

A common misconception is that disease risk is all in our genes: We are merely passengers on a time bomb waiting to happen. In reality, only a very small percentage of chronic diseases are inevitable. Less than 2 percent of all breast cancers are attributed to genetics. Similar numbers exist for other types of cancer, such as colon cancer, as well as heart disease, adult-onset diabetes, high blood pressure, and other degenerative disorders. Granted, certain genes might indicate a possible risk for a disease, but the effects of that gene only increase a person's susceptibility to the disease, they don't cause it. It's the combination of genetics and lifestyle that swings the pendulum from health to disease.

Our bodies have amazing defenses against disease, which evolved over millions of years and are finely tuned to combat most germs, chemicals, disease processes, and even aging itself. If our defenses were provided with all the building blocks necessary to do their jobs, it's likely that most bodies would live relatively disease free and robustly well into advanced years. These defense systems include the antioxidants, the immune system, cell communication, and apoptosis.

THE ANTI-DISEASE SYSTEM

Oxygen is our most important nutrient. But while 95 percent of the oxygen we breathe goes to life-giving processes, the remaining fraction comes packaged as oxygen fragments called free radicals. These highly reactive compounds enter the body in food, air, and from normal metabolic processes. They attack cell membranes, proteins, and even the cells' genetic code, damaging cells in much the same way that air causes fats to go rancid, rubber to lose its elasticity, and iron to rust. At a rate of ten thousand free radical "tears" in your body's cells each day, this equates to millions of tears over the course of a lifetime. If even 1 percent of the oxygen we breathed every day contained free radicals, that would equate to two kilograms per year! It is this backlog of cellular damage that contributes to the aging process and its associated diseases.

Free radicals aren't all bad. Our ancient ancestors counted on free radicals to produce mutations that probably helped advance our species. Free radicals also acted much like the first antibiotics by killing harmful germs. However, left unchecked in today's lifestyles, this inherent ability to mutate contributes to all major degenerative diseases. Free radicals contribute to the initiation and progression of most cancers. They damage the carriers of cholesterol in the blood, called lipoproteins, increasing their stickiness and promoting the progression of atherosclerosis. Free radicals damage artery walls, as well as worsen tissue damage during heart attack and stroke. They damage proteins in the lens of the eye, resulting in cataracts. They contribute to the progression of diabetes, arthritis, memory loss and Alzheimer's disease, Parkinson's disease, kidney failure, inflammation and inflammatory bowel syndrome, rheumatoid arthritis, AIDS, lupus, ALS, and even premature aging. Were it not for evolution, we wouldn't last long around free radicals.

When algae first began manufacturing oxygen, this noxious gas killed many primitive life forms that had thrived in an oxygen-free environment. Those that survived and evolved developed a defense to protect themselves against oxygen toxicity. This ancient defense, including a complex system of anti-free-radical enzymes, phytochemicals, and nutrients such as vitamin C, beta carotene, and vitamin E, is called our antioxidant system. It allows us to thrive on oxygen.

Fighting off oxygen fragments required a hefty dose of antioxidants, which were supplied in our evolutionary diets. It's no wonder that thousands of studies show that antioxidant-rich diets prevent disease and premature aging. Antioxidants also help maintain and stimulate the immune system, thus protecting the body from disease and infection that can lead to premature death. People with high blood antioxidant levels comparable to those maintained by our ancient ancestors have the lowest rates of heart disease, cancer, cataracts, and numerous other diseases. They also live longer.

A FORTRESS UNDER SIEGE

Since the dawn of creation, our bodies have been like fortresses under constant attack. Everything in the environment—from the air they breathed to the animals and other people they met—constantly exposed our ancient ancestors to bacteria, viruses, and other germs with the potential to cause infection or disease. If our ancestors hadn't developed immune systems to combat the onslaught, we wouldn't be here today. While your antioxidant system is sweeping up free radicals, a well-functioning immune system correctly recognizes a foreign invader, multiplies its forces, destroys the enemy, calls off the troops, and creates memory cells that file data on future invaders.

Our ancient ancestors had powerful immune systems. For example, researchers at the University of Notre Dame report no signs of meningitis in ancient foragers. Granted, infectious disease escalated with the development of agriculture, in part because of increased crowding. But the immune system also weakened when we strayed from our evolutionary roots by eating poor diets, not effectively coping with chronic stress, smoking, and being sedentary. The result is chronic or repeated infections, serious illnesses such as cancer, and an increased likelihood of dying prematurely.

CELL COMMUNICATION

Cells talk. Not with words, but they signal back and forth to coordinate and control their growth and the growth of neighboring cells. Much of this system depends on cell-to-cell channels called gap junctions, which are water-filled pores in cell membranes that connect adjoining cells. Through these pores flows constant information on how the cell is growing and whether or not damaging substances are present. This constant cell-to-cell communication helps the body identify the presence of abnormal cell growth or cancer, the beginnings of atherosclerosis, and the state of the union in a developing baby.

CELL SUICIDE

Programmed cell death (called apoptosis) is another way cells protect themselves from disease. When a cell damaged by free radicals, heat, radiation, or toxic chemicals cannot repair itself, or in the case of cancer grows out of control, mechanisms within the cell speed its death. This allows the body to eliminate large numbers of damaged cells without triggering inflammation or further damage to neighboring tissues. Apoptosis of abnormal cells reduces the growth and spread of disease. On the other hand, suppression of apoptosis increases cancer growth, infection, and the progression of other degenerative diseases, as well as premature aging.

Our diets help regulate apoptosis. A nutrient-poor diet speeds apoptosis of healthy cells (and therefore encourages disease and aging). An optimal diet slows apoptosis of healthy cells and helps the body destroy abnormal cells. Calorie restriction, as in the case of short-term fasts, also enhances apoptosis of damaged cells, which might explain why cutting back on unnecessary calories reduces disease risk and prolongs life. (See more on calorie restriction later in this chapter.)

WHY DO DEFENSES BREAK DOWN?

With such a diverse array of protective systems, how and why do we get sick? The answer to that question is complex and poorly understood. However, research shows that diet plays a critical role in maintaining the body's natural defenses against disease. For example, our ancestors evolved on diets rich in the antioxidant nutrients, especially vitamin C, beta carotene, and the phytochemicals. After the introduction of agriculture, diets supplied fewer antioxidant-rich plants, and defense systems dependent on those nutrients suffered.

Today, only one out of every one hundred people consume diets that meet even minimum standards for adequacy. People who consume optimal diets or who supplement good diets with extra antioxidants significantly boost their antioxidant defense systems, enhance immune function, and speed apoptosis in abnormal cells. Beta carotene is also essential for normal cell-to-cell communication, yet we consume only a fraction of the beta carotene found in ancient diets.

These systems work in concert, so a dietary deficiency that affects one system, such as the antioxidant system, has a domino effect on the other defenses. It's no surprise that numerous nutrients in abundance in ancient diets—from vitamins E, B_6, C, and D to magnesium, chromium, calcium, and zinc—are low in the diets of people today who are at risk for developing diabetes, heart disease, cancer, and other chronic conditions. To compound the issue, air pollution, fried foods, pesticides, cigarette smoke, and chronic stress increase our exposure to free radicals to levels unprecedented in pre-agricultural times. Our natural defense systems are taxed like never before.

Other aspects of our evolutionary lives also kept these defense systems humming in harmony. Daily moderate exercise, effective coping with stress, avoiding tobacco, and including relaxation time in the daily schedule boost the immune system and our resistance to colds, infections, and disease. In short, living in tune with our ancient inheritance helps the body run smoothly, in harmony and balance, and free of disease.

WHY AREN'T WE ALL SICK?

Some people are at higher risk for disease because of lifestyle choices and genetic quirks. Since the development of agriculture, humans have been living in a world unfamiliar to our 100,000-plus genes. Natural selection cannot change our body design fast enough to cope with these rapid changes. Each of us has a slightly different evolutionary history with a slightly different genetic blueprint, so it's not surprising that genetic quirks that went unnoticed in pre-agricultural times become major health problems, such as diabetes or heart disease, for some people in today's novel environment. These quirks aren't defects; they were harmless or maybe even helpful in ancient times. They just don't mesh well when combined with current diets, activity levels, and lifestyles.

Our Ancestors Ate Their Medicine

Most of the major diseases in westernized societies—including heart disease, cancer, hypertension, and diabetes—are caused by living out of sync with our evolutionary roots. For example:

• Our ancient ancestors were lean. Today, skyrocketing obesity rates increase the risk for developing chronic diseases. The more overweight people are, the greater their risks.

• Our ancestors were fit. Today, inactive lifestyles encourage weight gain, elevate blood fats, reduce blood sugar regulation, and increase the risk for depression, osteoporosis, memory loss, fatigue, and a host of other emotional and physical problems.

• Our ancestors ate antioxidant-rich diets. Today, our diets are low in antioxidants, while all of the major diseases are related to free radical damage and inadequate antioxidant systems.

• Our Paleolithic ancestors didn't smoke and they worked off their stress. Today, tobacco use, inactivity, and chronic stress escalate disease risk.

- Our ancestors ate low-fat, high-fiber foods. Today's diets are high in fat, sugar, salt, and saturated fat and low in fiber, fruits, vegetables, and calcium, all of which increase disease risk.

The good news is that most of the diseases of affluence can be prevented. For example, up to 70 percent of all cancers are a result of lifestyle; the vast majority of diabetics could be free from their disease just by losing excess body weight; and heart disease and hypertension are preventable, curable, and even reversible by making better choices about what you eat, when you move, and how you live. Here's why living in tune with your ancient past could keep you healthy and vital well past one hundred years of age.

Eat More Produce

Our bodies evolved on three to four pounds of produce every day. Today we consume a few ounces. "If the only dietary change people make is to eat more fruits and vegetables, a number of other dietary issues will fall into line," recommends Susan Krebs-Smith, Ph.D., R.D., research nutritionist for the National Cancer Institute in Bethesda, Maryland.

Hundreds of studies spanning decades of research show that diets brimming with fruits and vegetables help you lose weight, live longer, and reduce your risk for heart disease, stroke, cancer, diabetes, hypertension, cataracts, and possibly arthritis. The effects are astonishing!

- Cancer risk alone drops by half just by doubling the current intake of produce.
- Blood cholesterol levels drop 33 percent in just two weeks when women boost their intakes of produce.
- Risk for bronchitis, ulcers, gallstones, cirrhosis, kidney stones, arthritis, and cancers of the lungs, stomach, esophagus, mouth, endometrium, pancreas, cervix, colon, urinary tract, and possibly breast also drop dramatically when people eat more fruits and vegetables.

• Raise fruit and vegetable intakes to levels eaten by our ancient ancestors and blood pressures drop in patients with hypertension as dramatically as they do with drug treatment.

That's just the beginning of the health benefits. A study from Tufts University in Boston found that women eating the most fruits and vegetables also had the least bone loss and the lowest risk for osteoporosis. Fruits and vegetables also might be the fountain of youth. In 1998, researchers from the University of Naples in Italy studied people from the ages of seventy to more than one hundred years and found that those living the longest also were living the healthiest. Their secret? They ate lots more fruits and vegetables than their younger, less healthy friends.

Our bodies thrive on fresh produce for a number of reasons. Fruits and vegetables

1. have no fat, cholesterol, or sodium (with the exception of avocados, olives, and coconuts);

2. are some of the most fiber-rich foods in the diet (eight servings of fruits and vegetables daily supplies approximately 27 grams of fiber, well within the daily target goal of 25 to 35 grams);

3. are packed with nutrients, supplying ample amounts of calcium, iron, magnesium, and health-promoting vitamins such as folic acid. Our bodies evolved expecting high levels of these nutrients. Without optimal intakes, we develop osteoporosis, anemia, diabetes, heart disease, cancer, cataracts, arthritis, and other disorders; and

4. are low in calories. They average as little as one calorie per gram, compared to up to nine calories per gram in highly refined foods.

Most of the foods on our ancient ancestors' plates were plants. So it's no wonder that no other food is so closely linked to lifelong health and longevity. What our ancestors did out of necessity and our grandparents told us to do out of love, we must now do out of enlightened self-interest—triple our current intakes of fruits and vegetables!

PHYTOCHEMICAL WONDERS

Nutritionally speaking, there's more to fruits and vegetables than vitamins, minerals, and fiber. Thousands of other compounds in these foods, called phytochemicals or plant nutrients, pack an extra health-enhancing punch.

For example, the bioflavonoids in citrus fruits and vegetables reduce blood clots associated with stroke and inhibit the oxidation of cholesterol that turns harmless fats in the blood into the sticky glue that clogs artery walls. Sulforaphane in broccoli is an antioxidant that bolsters the body's natural defense mechanisms against cancer. Lutein in spinach prevents normal cells from converting to abnormal cells by improving cell-to-cell communication. The hundreds of sulfur compounds in garlic also might slow the hands of time. "Garlic appears to have a beneficial effect in stimulating immune function and lowering blood cholesterol levels even when consumed in moderate amounts of one to one and a half cloves a day," says Dr. Jeffrey Blumberg. The list of phytochemicals is endless and grows daily as researchers uncover more of these health-enhancing plant nutrients. (See The Anti-Cancer Army in Vegetables and Fruits below for a list of some of these compounds.)

THE ANTI-CANCER ARMY IN VEGETABLES AND FRUITS

Mother Nature packed nutritional muscle into fruits and vegetables. In addition to hefty doses of antioxidant nutrients such as vitamins C and E and selenium, folic acid, and fiber, vegetables and fruit contain more than 12,000 compounds that boost your body's natural defenses against disease. They encourage cells to raise their levels of enzymes that hinder cancer-causing substances from initiating cancer, act as antioxidants to fend off cancer, and regulate hormones that otherwise encourage cancer growth. Here's a partial list of what you'll find on a plateful of plants.

- Allium compounds, such as diallyl sulfide and allyl methyl trisulfide, in garlic, chives, leeks, and onions

- Carotinoids, such as alpha and beta carotene, lutein, lycopene, and capsanthin, in deep-colored produce, paprika
- Coumarins in tea, soybeans, cruciferous vegetables, citrus, and flaxseed
- Flavonoids, such as anthocyanidins, catechins, flavonones, and flavones, in fruit, vegetables, citrus, and tea
- Indoles, such as indole-3-carbinol, in cabbage, broccoli, Brussels sprouts, and other cruciferous vegetables
- Inositol hexaphosphate, in whole grains and legumes
- Isoflavones, such as genistein, diadzein, and biochanin A, in whole wheat and soybeans
- Isothiocyanates, such as sulforaphane and PEITC, in cruciferous vegetables, turnips, and watercress
- Phenols and polyphenols, such as caffeic acid, ferulic acid, quercetin, and ellagic acid, in oats, soybeans, blueberries, prunes, grapes, and strawberries
- Phytoestrogens, such as lignans and the isoflavones diadzein and genistein, in soybeans, flax, rye, and vegetables
- Phytosterols, such as beta-sitosterol, stigmasterol, and campesterol, in legumes
- Probiotics and prebiotics, such as fructo-oligosaccharides and *Lactobacillus,* in Jerusalem artichokes, shallots, yogurt, and soybeans
- Saponins, such as spirostan and furostan, in legumes
- Tannins, such as proanthrocyanidins, in cranberries, tea, and chocolate
- Terpenes, such as D-limonene, in citrus fruits

Fiber Up

Our evolutionary diets contained 100 to 150 grams of fiber. Today we average closer to 10 to 20 grams. Returning to our original fiber intakes is one of the easiest ways to bring our health back in balance with our heritage, lower our disease risk, and reduce our waistlines.

According to researchers at the Harvard School of Public Health, heart-disease risk drops 20 percent for every 10 grams of fiber added to our diets. Fiber lowers heart-disease risk by lowering LDL and total cholesterol, triglycerides, blood pressure, and obesity. It helps flush bile acids from the body, thus lowering the body's pool of excess cholesterol. Fiber also speeds the removal of potential cancer-causing substances, thus lowering colon cancer risk. Fiber-rich foods slow the absorption of glucose, preventing wide swings in blood sugar and helping lower diabetes risk. The health benefits are endless. While disease risk increases in proportion to the amount of refined grains in people's diets, risk decreases as intake of fiber-rich whole grains increases.

The benefits of fiber come primarily from eating a wide variety of whole foods, not a smattering of highly refined bran products. It's whole foods that our ancestors ate and that are packed with other health-enhancing nutrients and phytochemicals (including the anti-cancer compound inositol hexaphosphate), as well as the wide assortment of fibers. William Connor, M.D., professor in the School of Medicine at Oregon Health Sciences University in Portland and lead researcher of the Family Heart Study, adds, "If people obtained most of their calories from whole foods, such as fruits, vegetables, whole grains, and legumes, they would be well on their way to good health."

GRANDMA CALLED IT ROUGHAGE

Fiber is an umbrella term for a wide variety of insoluble and soluble fibers. The insoluble fibers in whole grains and vegetables absorb water in the digestive tract, increase stool bulk, speed the movement of waste products through the digestive tract, and help prevent colon cancer, constipation, diverticulosis, irritable bowel syndrome, and hemorrhoids. The soluble fibers, such as the vegetable gums and pectin, are found in fruits, cooked dried beans and peas, and oats. They help curb erratic swings in blood sugar levels and lower blood cholesterol, thus helping prevent or treat diabetes and cardiovascular disease.

The Fiber Scoreboard: High-Fiber Foods

The following foods are high in fiber (3 grams or more of fiber per serving) and low in fat.

	AMOUNT	FIBER (GRAMS)
Bulgur (cracked wheat)	1 cup cooked	8.1
Whole wheat spaghetti	1 cup cooked	5.9
Whole wheat couscous	1 cup cooked	3.9
Popcorn, air-popped	3 cups	3.9
Brown rice	1 cup cooked	3.3
Whole grain waffles	2	3.0
		(plus 2 grams fat)
Wheat bran	½ cup	12.6
Rice bran	⅓ cup	6.1
Oat bran	⅔ cup	4.0
Pinto beans	¾ cup cooked	14.2
Kidney beans	¾ cup cooked	13.8
Black-eyed peas	¾ cup cooked	12.3
Baked potato, with skin	1 medium	4.2
Sweet potato, without skin	1 medium	3.4
Brussels sprouts	½ cup cooked	3.3
Salsa, homemade	½ cup	3.0
Figs, dried	3	5.3
Guava	1	5.3
Pear	1	4.3
Apricots, dried	10	3.6
Prunes, dried	5	3.5
Orange	1	3.1
Almonds	¼ cup	3.8
Pistachios	¼ cup	3.8

THE GLYCEMIC ISSUE

The glycemic index is a measure (from 0 to 100) of how rapidly and dramatically blood sugar levels rise after eating a particular food. Foods with high glycemic scores spike blood sugar levels, while low glycemic foods produce modest rises in blood sugar. Elevated blood sugar, in turn, contributes to diabetes risk. In fact, people who eat the least amount of fiber and the most high-glycemic foods have a 2½ times greater risk for developing diabetes than do people who eat closer to their evolutionary roots.

Most high-glycemic foods, such as highly processed grains, instant and processed foods, sweets, and potatoes, are also foods alien to ancient diets. Although the glycemic score for a potato is 100, more ancient roots such as sweet potatoes or yams score under 50. Refined grains probably spike blood sugar levels because they lack the fiber in whole grains that slows absorption and produces a gentle release of glucose into the bloodstream.

Research repeatedly finds that eating foods from our past reduces diabetes risk. David Jenkins, Ph.D., at the University of Toronto, found that blood sugar levels were lowest in diabetics fed whole grains, while blood sugar levels rose as whole grain consumption decreased. He concluded that the large particle size of the whole grain helped lower blood sugar, while this protective effect was lost when grains were processed. In short, people prone to diabetes do well returning to a more ancient diet based on minimally processed foods with low glycemic scores.

Granted, people who quickly convert from a high-fat, low-fiber diet to one lower in fat and higher in carbohydrates often experience a temporary elevation in blood triglyceride levels. The body adapts, however, and triglycerides drop within about twelve weeks of adopting this healthier eating style. You can curb the triglyceride rise by gradually increasing carbohydrates, while cutting back on fat, and by eating whole grains instead of refined grains.

BEANS FOR BREAKFAST, BEANS FOR DINNER

Legumes were a part of our heritage. Supplying more than nine grams of fiber per serving, these are nature's best source of fiber, as well as excellent sources of protein, B vitamins, and minerals. Beans put domesticated meat to shame, lowering blood cholesterol, strengthening bones,

The Glycemic Index: Modern versus Ancient Foods

The glycemic index ranks foods according to how quickly and dramatically they raise blood sugar levels, with 100 being the highest score. Some high-fiber foods receive a high ranking, but that doesn't mean they're off limits. These foods, such as carrots, parsnips, and whole wheat bread, rank high because they are low in soluble fiber, which is the best type of fiber for curbing blood sugar levels. These foods are excellent sources of insoluble fibers, which protect the colon from cancer, constipation, hemorrhoids, and other digestive tract problems.

FOOD	GLYCEMIC INDEX (%)
Glucose	100
Parsnips	97
Carrots	92
Honey	87
Corn flakes, instant potatoes	80
Whole wheat bread, white rice	72
White bread	69
Candy bar	68
Shredded wheat	67
Brown rice	66
Beets	64
Buckwheat, green peas, yams	51
Oatmeal	49
Sweet potato	48
Whole wheat spaghetti noodles	42
Oranges	40
Legumes (cooked dried beans, lentils, peas)	29–40*
Apples	39
Soybeans	15

*Depending on the bean.

and possibly boosting immunity. They also are phytochemical power-houses, loaded with saponins that lower blood cholesterol levels, phyto-sterols that lower colon-cancer risk, and protease inhibitors that slow tumor growth.

Soybeans contain phytoestrogens that boost immunity, help keep blood vessels flexible, and block estrogen from entering cells, thus reducing the risk for hormone-related cancers such as ovarian, prostate, and breast cancers. These weak estrogen-like compounds also buffer estrogen swells, which possibly curb hot flashes and other symptoms of menopause. According to Mark Messina, future research will investigate their usefulness in a variety of other conditions, from treating alcoholism and boosting brain function to managing middle-age spread and hyper-tension, and preventing cataracts.

No Man-Made Pesticides

Our food supply is laced with thousands of synthetic pesticides, and no one has a clear idea of the damage they cause to human health. One thing is for sure: Man-made pesticides were absent for 99.9 percent of the time humans have been on earth.

We know that some pesticides alter the health and reproductive success of wildlife and their offspring. Although most researchers doubt that the low levels of environmental pesticides are high enough to cause similar health effects in humans, that's really just an educated guess. The Environmental Protection Agency reports that approximately seventy pesticides now in use are probable or possible cancer-causing agents. In addition, we have no natural inclination to avoid these novel toxins. Evolution equipped us with the ability to taste and smell common natural toxins and the motivation to avoid these bitter or vile-smelling compounds. But modern pesticides are odorless, tasteless, and too new for our bodies to have evolved avoidance responses.

On the other hand, some researchers believe the pesticide scare is more smoke than fire. According to Dr. Bruce Ames at the University of

California, Berkeley, our bodies evolved elaborate defenses against environmental toxins. For example, our digestive tracts regularly shed their lining, many enzymes detoxify dangerous chemicals from the environment, diarrhea quickly eliminates unwanted substances, and antioxidants combat toxic free radicals. These defenses are generalists, not specialists, so it makes good evolutionary sense that they would work against both natural and synthetic compounds.

The pesticide issue should be placed in perspective. We ingest approximately ten thousand times more natural pesticides than man-made chemicals. For example, we consume canavanine in alfalfa sprouts, hydrazines in raw mushrooms, and other carcinogens in herb teas. Cooking destroys some of these natural toxins, but creates others, such as nitrosamines and nitropyrenes formed when meat is cooked. Dr. Ames states that eliminating the small amount of synthetic chemicals in our diets would have no effect on cancer rates, and that exposure to pesticides is nowhere near as important a health concern as smoking, excessive alcohol consumption, being overweight, or consuming too much saturated fat.

Does organic produce have lower levels of synthetic pesticides, and is it better for us? Most reports that organic produce is healthier than conventional produce are anecdotal. However, a literature review on organic agricultural methods from the past fifty years conducted at NutriKenetics in Washington, D.C., found that organic produce might have slightly higher concentrations of vitamin C, lower levels of nitrate, and higher protein quality compared to conventional produce. In addition, studies on animals show better growth and reproduction in animals fed organically grown feed. These benefits result from more than just the absence of pesticides and indicate a fundamental difference between organic and chemical fertilizers and fertility-enhancing effects. No studies exist to show whether or not organic versus conventional foods are healthier for humans.

Regardless of the pesticide controversy, fresh, unprocessed foods were some of the most nutritious foods in our ancient ancestors' diets, and are the food on which our bodies evolved. They should be eaten in greater quantities even if they have traces of man-made pesticides. Ways to reduce pesticide exposure will be covered in chapter 5.

Good Fat—Bad Fat

Wild game is low in saturated fat and high in omega-3 fatty acids. Domesticated meat, as well as fatty dairy products (cheese, whole milk, cream cheese, sour cream), are just the reverse: high in saturated fat and low in omega-3s. Our bodies have not adapted well to the switch from omega-3s to saturated fat, just as our cars would run poorly if we fueled them with grease instead of gasoline.

How Fat Intake Compares to Heart Disease Risk

Increases in the total saturated fat intake, as well as the ratio of saturated fat to omega-3s, have caused a rapid increase in heart disease risk.

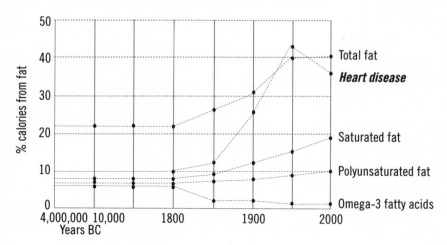

There's a big difference between the omega-3s and saturated fat. The omega-3s are structural fats used by the body to build cell membranes, regulate nerve activity, and monitor bone formation. Saturated fats are storage fats that are either used for energy or deposited into fat tissues or onto artery walls. Tampering with these fundamental fats has escalated our risks for heart disease, diabetes, inflammatory disorders, cancer, obesity, schizophrenia, aggressiveness and hostility, and even attention deficit disorder, Alzheimer's disease, suicide, lupus, arthritis, and allergies (the latter also might result from our unnatural indoor living, especially with wall-to-wall carpeting that harbors dust mites). Very low intakes of omega-3s result in numbness, tingling, weakness, leg pain, and blurred vision.

OMEGA-3S AND HEALTH

Fatty fish is the best source of omega-3s these days. People who regularly include salmon, mackerel, or other fatty fish in their diets are less likely to die prematurely. For example, researchers at the Catholic University in Leuven, Belgium, obtained information from the Food and Agriculture Organization and the World Health Organization that compared fish consumption to all causes of death in thirty-six countries. Results showed that the more fish people consumed the less likely they were to die from any cause, but especially heart disease and stroke. People cut their risk by half when they consumed at least an ounce or two of fish daily.

New research suggests that how smart you are, your mood, and even your risk for osteoporosis might also depend on your intake of these fats. The omega-3s function at the very foundation of many body processes, turning on and off the immune system and hormonelike compounds called prostaglandins that regulate such diverse processes as bone formation, pain tolerance, sleep, body temperature, appetite, and artery wall function. As components of cell membranes, the omega-3s decide what comes and goes from cells, thus regulating neurotransmitter activity and tissue development, including vision and brain capacity. These fats even help regulate what enters and leaves the brain. For example, a deficiency of these fats in diabetes interferes with the transfer of sugar into the brain.

Until recently, preventing osteoporosis focused only on calcium. But that is likely to change as researchers such as Bruce Watkins, Ph.D., professor of food science at Purdue University, delve deeper into how to influence the fundamental mechanisms that stimulate bone cells to build tissue. In his studies, Dr. Watkins found that the omega-3s turn on prostaglandin production, which triggers bone cells to deposit calcium. Omega-3s also help boost calcium absorption and enhance the action of vitamin D in bone building. Our bodies evolved on diets that contained ample calcium and omega-3s, which explains why osteoporosis was unknown in those ultra-ancient times.

OMEGA-3S, DEPRESSION, AND SANITY

"My mood is great, more even, and I feel better, too!" said Natalie.

"I feel great! My energy level and mood are good and constant, not high and low, throughout the day, so I don't have to push myself after lunch," added LeRoy.

"By the second week of being on the Origin Diet, I turned the corner on energy. I'm waking up with a lot more energy, sleeping better, feel more alert and less stressed. I don't hit the slumps like I used to and my moods are more level," says Patricia.

Those words are heard time and again by people who have switched from their typical American diets to the Origin Diet. One reason for the mood boost could be the high levels of omega-3s.

As mentioned above, the omega-3s constitute one third of our brains and are important regulators of brain function. In fact, many researchers suspect that it was the rise in intakes of omega-3s that led to the evolution of our large brains. Today, we consume a fraction of the omega-3s that were in our ancient ancestors' diets, and depression rates have increased hundredfold, rating as the number-one cause of disability in some Western societies.

Limit intake of these fats and brain function, thinking ability, mood, and behavior are affected. Preliminary studies from the National Institute on Alcohol Abuse and Alcoholism in Rockville, Maryland, show that increasing intakes of omega-3s might boost serotonin activity and help curb depression, impulsive violence, and even suicide. In contrast, cultures where people consume low amounts of omega-3s have the world's highest incidence of these problems. The omega-3s also might

MOOD BOOSTERS

Battling the blues? Feeling cranky? It could be your diet. People who adopt the Origin Diet report that they feel better, have more energy, and sleep better. Here are six habits they adopt as part of the Origin Diet to boost their moods:

- Habit 1: Make sure every meal contains wholesome, complex carbohydrates. Plan a carbohydrate-rich snack, such as whole grain crackers and peanut butter or baked tortilla chips and low-fat bean dip, to curb midafternoon snack attacks.
- Habit 2: Cut out sugar, including desserts, sugar-coated cereals, candy, sugar-sweetened beverages, and sugary snack foods such as granola bars. Work with sweet cravings by replacing refined sweets with ancient sweets, such as a whole grain bagel with honey or plain low-fat yogurt sweetened with fresh fruit.
- Habit 3: Cut back on caffeine from coffee, tea, chocolate, cocoa, colas, and medications. Drink more water.
- Habit 4: Increase your intake of vitamin-B_6-rich foods, such as chicken breast, legumes, fish, bananas, avocados, whole grains, and dark green leafy vegetables. Also include at least two folic-acid-rich foods in the diet daily, such as spinach, broccoli, orange juice, or chard.
- Habit 5: Make changes gradually. Select two or three small changes and practice these until they are comfortable. This will assure long-term success in sticking with your plan and will allow your brain chemistry time to adjust to the new eating style, without throwing your nerve chemicals into a tailspin.
- Habit 6: Take a moderate-dose multiple vitamin and mineral supplement to fill in any nutritional gaps.

have helped our ancient ancestors stay sane. In a study from Brigham and Women's Hospital in Boston, researchers found that omega-3s acted as mood stabilizers in people undergoing treatment for manic depression. In another study on patients with bipolar disorder, relapse rates dropped from 52 percent to 12 percent when patients supplemented with the omega-3s.

Our bodies evolved on other fats in addition to the omega-3s. All of these fats also help maintain the body's natural defenses against disease. For example, the fats found in olive oil, avocados, and nuts reduce the risk for heart disease, cancer, and premature death. Nuts might even help people lose weight. It's the new fats, such as high doses of saturated fat, the trans fatty acids in processed foods, and the hefty doses of processed oils that are unfamiliar to our evolved bodies and that increase disease risk, contribute to high obesity rates, and undermine longevity.

NO TRANS FATTY ACIDS

Trans fatty acids (TFAs) were probably found in ultra-ancient diets, but in tiny amounts. Hydrogenating vegetable oils to make margarine and shortening has dramatically increased our intakes of these fats. "The worst thing that happened to our diets is that natural fats were pulled out and replaced with large amounts of hydrogenated vegetable oils," says Mary Enig, Ph.D., former research associate at the University of Maryland and one of the first researchers to investigate TFAs in our food. (See chapter 2 for a detailed description of TFAs.)

According to Dr. Enig, TFAs increase our risk for everything from heart disease and diabetes to infertility and reduced resistance to colds and disease. Walter Willett, M.D., Dr.P.H., and colleagues at the Harvard School of Public Health in Boston compared dietary intakes to disease rates in more than 85,000 women and found that as intakes of TFA-containing foods, including margarine, cookies, biscuits, and cakes, increased, so did women's risks for heart disease. Dr. Willett believes that TFAs contribute to 30,000 heart disease deaths in the United States each year. "We are not yet sure about the exact magnitude of the issue. Certainly trans fatty acid intake has less of an effect [on heart disease risk] than does smoking or lack of physical activity and probably a similar effect as a high saturated fat intake," says Dr. Willett.

Milk Tolerance

Our ancestors consumed about 1,900 milligrams of calcium daily and showed no signs of osteoporosis. Today, women average only about 600 milligrams; 20 million women over the age of forty suffer from this bone disease. "Women's calcium needs are greater than we previously thought and may be as much as four to five times higher than they are getting from their diets," says Robert P. Heaney, M.D., a calcium expert and John A. Creighton University Professor at Creighton University in Omaha. High calcium intakes prevent osteoporosis and since few people get enough calcium, research has focused on supplements. As Dr. Heaney says, "The strongest evidence is with calcium supplements; however, several studies in the past few years have used milk products as a calcium source and have found similar benefits."

Milk is a relatively modern part of our diets, gracing tables only after animals were domesticated a few thousand years ago. Does that mean we shouldn't drink milk? This is one area where Stone Age conflicts with "New" Age. "It is very difficult to meet calcium requirements when milk is avoided, because there are so few foods as rich in calcium that people are willing to eat frequently," states Bess Dawson-Hughes, chief of the Calcium and Bone Metabolism Laboratory at the USDA Human Nutrition Research Center on Aging at Tufts University in Boston. Other calcium-rich sources include dark green leafy vegetables and beans, which were in our ancestors' primary sources, but it takes 25 cups of raw broccoli, 10 cups of cooked chard, or 21 cups of kidney beans to get even 1,000 milligrams of calcium. One reasonable alternative is calcium-fortified soymilk or calcium-fortified orange juice.

You can take calcium pills, but this goes against the common sense recommendation to turn first to food and only to supplements as a last resort. "There is no evidence that calcium supplements are better than milk for preventing osteoporosis, and food always should be the first choice for obtaining optimal nutrition," says Dawson-Hughes. Milk also contains vitamin D, a deficiency of which results in poor calcium absorption and rapid bone loss. In fact, Dr. Dawson–Hughes's research shows that increasing vitamin D intake, even in people with adequate calcium intake, can help reduce bone fractures and slow the progression of osteoporosis.

Where Else Can You Get Calcium?

Milk supplies up to 75 percent of an adult's need for calcium, a mineral essential for maintaining optimal health and preventing osteoporosis, hypertension, and colon cancer. It requires careful planning to get enough calcium if this food group is eliminated from the diet. The following food servings are comparable in calcium content to a glass of milk (i.e., approximately 300 milligrams). Most adults need between 1,000 milligrams and 1,200 milligrams of calcium daily.

FOOD	SERVING SIZE
Broccoli, cooked	3 cups
Mustard greens, cooked	1½ cups
Collard greens, cooked	1 cup
Oysters	1½ cups
Canned salmon with bones	5 ounces
Orange	5 medium
Dried beans, cooked	3 cups
Spinach, cooked	1¼ cups
Dandelion greens, cooked	1 cup
Soymilk*	30 cups

*Soymilk contains only 10 milligrams of calcium per cup, unless it is calcium fortified.

DOES MILK MAKE YOU SICK?

Claims that milk causes heart disease are based on epidemiological studies that compared the heart disease risk and milk consumption rates of different countries. Sure enough, those countries, such as Finland, where people drank the most milk, also had the highest rates of heart disease. According to Dr. Heaney, the only true link between milk and heart disease is with the saturated fat. With an abundance of nonfat milk, yogurt, and cheese products on the market, you can easily meet your calcium needs without sacrificing your heart.

Milk also doesn't cause diabetes. A few preliminary studies found a link between a series of amino acids in cow's milk, called ABBOS, and juvenile onset diabetes in children with a genetic predisposition to the disease. The studies suggested that when these children ingest ABBOS, it triggers an immune response that attacks the milk protein and the insulin-producing cells in the pancreas. Over time, the cells are destroyed and the child becomes diabetic. However, the evidence linking milk to diabetes is inconclusive. In fact, the only real proof is that breast-feeding is protective against the development of diabetes, not that cow's milk or formulas made with cow's milk are necessarily harmful.

If there is a link between cow's milk and diabetes it is most likely only in babies under one year old whose digestive tracts are still permeable, allowing large chunks of proteins like ABBOS to enter the blood and set off a reaction. It's not earthshaking news to hear that babies shouldn't drink cow's milk; since 1976, the American Academy of Pediatrics has warned against feeding cow's milk to infants. There is no solid evidence yet that anyone other than the under-one set, even children and adults genetically at risk for diabetes, is harmed by drinking milk—that is, unless they are milk intolerant.

The only real problem with milk is for those people who are lactose intolerant (see the box on page 87 to find out if you are). These people lack the enzyme to break down lactose, or milk sugar, and develop gas and intestinal cramping when they drink milk. While milk allergy receives a lot of attention, it is rarely diagnosed in adults. The 1 to 2 percent of young children who develop allergic symptoms to milk, including bronchitis, eczema, and asthma, usually outgrow the problem by the time they are two years old. Even people who are lactose intolerant can often drink small amounts of milk with meals or can eat yogurt (the ones made with the bacteria *Lactobacillus bulgaricus* or possibly *Lactobacillus acidophilus* are the best) or drink nonfat milk treated with lactase, such as Lactaid.

ARE YOU INTOLERANT?

Without enough of the digestive enzyme lactase, milk sugar is partially broken down by bacteria in the gut to produce acids and gases that cause gas and intestinal cramping within thirty minutes to a few hours after consuming milk. Are you intolerant? Take this test to find out.

Answer "yes" or "no" to the following questions:

____1. Do you frequently experience gas; digestive tract discomfort, bloating, and cramps; or diarrhea?

____2. Do uncomfortable symptoms develop within thirty minutes to two hours after consuming milk products, such as milk, cheese, or ice cream?

____3. Do these symptoms lessen or disappear when you avoid milk products for a week or more?

____4. Does anyone else in your family (i.e., your grandparents, father or mother, brothers or sisters, or aunts or uncles) develop any of the above symptoms after eating milk products?

____5. Are you Asian, Jewish, native American, Hispanic, Arabic, or African-American?

____6. Did you first notice these symptoms during or immediately after a digestive tract disorder, such as the stomach flu or gastroenteritis?

There is no exact number of "yes" or "no" answers that will guarantee a diagnosis of lactose intolerance. However, the more "yes" answers, the more likely you are to be lactose intolerant. A "yes" answer to the first question alone is no guarantee of lactose intolerance, since these are symptoms of many other disorders. A "yes" to the sixth question suggests you may have developed a lactose intolerance secondary to some other digestive tract problem. If this is the case, the intolerance should gradually subside if you refrain from milk products while treating the underlying infection. Even if you suffer from all the symptoms linked to lactose intolerance, beware of diagnosing yourself. Similar symptoms also are signs of other, more serious conditions and should be checked by a physician.

Good Bugs

Foragers' lives were anything but clean. They probably ingested a million times more bacteria than we do. Evolution developed a way to use the germs in the daily diet, and today more than five hundred different species of bacteria, totaling hundreds of grams, live in our digestive tracts. Healthful bacteria aid digestion, protect against the overgrowth of harmful germs and fungi, manufacture some nutrients, such as vitamin K and biotin, and help protect against disease, from colon cancer to diarrhea and intestinal infections. Healthful bacteria also protect the lungs, skin, eyes, and other tissues. Our sanitized lives and food supply means we are exposed to far fewer germs, with the main dietary source of health-enhancing bacteria being fermented foods and yogurt.

Research has uncovered links between the live bacteria in yogurt, especially *Lactobacillus bulgaricus* or *L. acidophilus*, *Streptococcus thermophilus*, and *Bifidobacterium*, and lowered disease risk. Termed probiotics, meaning "for life," these good germs, like the helpful bacteria in our ancient ancestors' diets, increase the absorption of nutrients, alleviate the symptoms of lactose intolerance, and fight cancer growth. These bacteria wade past the stomach and settle and flourish in the intestinal tract. They crowd out or kill off disease-causing bacteria, produce natural antibiotics, and possibly switch off an enzyme that triggers colon cancer. They also might lower breast cancer and heart disease risk.

The Anti-aging Aspects of the Origin Diet

Throw out every image you have of aging. Just about everything we've assumed as the inevitable consequences of aging—from memory loss to escalating disease risks—results more from years of living out of sync with our evolutionary past than from age per se. "We don't usually think of our lives as a result of the ingredients we put into them, but what we eat, what supplements we take, and how much we exercise shape how and when we age and to what extent we enjoy the process of living," says Dr. Blumberg.

ANTIOXIDANTS TO PREVENT MEMORY LOSS AND AGING

As if you haven't heard enough about antioxidants lowering the risk of everything from heart disease and cancer to cataracts and arthritis! According to Dr. Blumberg, a wealth of new research shows that these free-radical fighters don't just halt the progression of age-related diseases, they might even slow the aging process itself, protecting the body from the free radical wear and tear associated with tissue damage and aging. Recent research from the University of Wisconsin shows that the free radicals generated when glucose combines with oxygen damage many structures in the cell, particularly the energy-generating units known as mitochondria, which might be an underlying cause of aging. Reduce the generation of free radicals or boost antioxidant defenses and you slow the aging process.

Twelve Foods That Rev Brain Power

It's the entire diet that counts when it comes to thinking clearly. But a few foods pack an extra nutritional punch for mental power.

WHAT?	WHY?
1. Orange juice	One of nature's best sources of vitamin C, one glass supplies 124 milligrams of this antioxidant and 75 micrograms of folic acid, a B vitamin essential to the prevention of memory loss. Orange juice is also a source of limonene and bioflavonoids, phytochemicals that activate detoxifying enzymes.
2. Legumes	One cup of cooked beans, peas, or lentils supplies about 2.5 milligrams of zinc and ample amounts of brain-boosters such as calcium, iron, magnesium, folic acid and other B vitamins, fiber, protein, and complex carbohydrates.
3. Bananas	This fruit is one of the few plants high in vitamin B_6, a nutrient essential for circulation, brain function, energy metabolism, and the regulation of mood, pain tolerance, and sleep.

WHAT?	WHY?
4. Prunes	This dried fruit supplies more antioxidant phytochemicals than any other plant food. It's also an excellent source of iron.
5. Salmon	When it comes to the omega-3s, you can't get much better than salmon. A four-ounce serving supplies 1.63 milligrams of these essential fats, plus a hefty dose of vitamin B_{12}, which is important for memory and brain function.
6. Spinach	Two cups of spinach salad supply half your day's need for folic acid, 3 milligrams of iron, and lots of beta carotene, calcium, selenium, and vitamin C, all for less than 25 calories.
7. Tofu	A half-cup serving of firm tofu supplies more than 13 milligrams of iron! It is also a low-fat, low-sodium, low-cost source of protein, B vitamins, calcium, magnesium, and zinc.
8. Wheat germ	A half-cup serving of toasted wheat germ supplies more than half of your daily magnesium needs, as well as husky amounts of vitamins (including 100 percent of your daily folic acid and 50 percent of your vitamin E), iron, zinc, and choline.
9. Avocado	One avocado supplies one fourth of your daily need for magnesium and more than half the folic acid, one fourth the vitamin A, and lots of B vitamins, iron, and trace minerals.
10. Water	The most important nutrient is the most forgotten, yet even mild dehydration can cause mental fatigue, while drinking more water could lower bladder-cancer risk by reducing concentrations of cancer-causing substances in urine and speeding their removal by increasing urination.

WHAT?	WHY?
11. Sweet potato	An ideal alternative to the potato, sweet potatoes are excellent sources of antioxidants, folic acid, magnesium, and B vitamins. Their glycemic index score is also much lower than the white potato's.
12. Nonfat yogurt	The calcium in yogurt helps reduce absorption of lead, a toxic metal that damages the nervous system. Yogurt is also a good source of B vitamins, magnesium, zinc, and protein and a great source of probiotic bacteria.

Memory is a good example. Two studies, one on animals from the USDA Human Nutrition Research Center on Aging at Tufts University in Boston and one on humans from the University of Hawaii, report that boosting antioxidant intake lessens age-related damage to the central nervous system, thus slowing age-related memory loss. Antioxidants, such as vitamin E, also might help slow the progression of Alzheimer's disease. In one study, patients with moderately severe Alzheimer's disease slowed the progression of their disease by supplementing with antioxidants. Future research will likely uncover even more profound effects on how antioxidants increase longevity.

Create a Famine, Prolong Your Life

Life was not always good for our ancestors. Natural catastrophes and weather often upset the abundant supply of wild game and plants, resulting in periods of famine. Our bodies evolved ways to handle this feast and famine and might actually require it for optimal health. If the abundance of research on animals showing that calorie restriction increases lifespan can be applied to people, then cutting your food intake by about 30 percent for the rest of your life is all it would take to make you the healthiest two-hundred-year-old in the neighborhood.

"Calorie restriction is the only dietary habit known in mammals to improve both average and maximal lifespan," says Dr. George Roth, chief of the Molecular Physiology and Genetics Section of the National Institute on Aging in Baltimore. Every little mammal the researchers have studied increases its lifespan from two- to fourfold when calorie intake was cut to 60 percent to 70 percent of what's called *ad libitum,* or 60 percent to 70 percent of what the animals usually eat to feel satisfied. The benefits of semi-fasting far exceed just living longer; the hungry animals are also relatively free from heart disease, diabetes, cancer, memory loss, and age-related loss of immune function. Blood levels of disease-causing free radicals also drop when calories are curtailed.

In evolutionary terms, it's likely that the effects of cutting back on calories did not evolve to increase lifespan, but to improve survival so humans could reproduce. Even so, the secret is undernutrition, not malnutrition, which means reducing calories while still providing all the vitamins and minerals in optimal amounts for health. That means cutting back on unnecessary calories, which come entirely from modern-day foods such as saturated fat, sugar, and alcohol, while focusing on foods typically found in ancient times.

While cutting calories by 30 percent is severe for most people, even a modest reduction—perhaps cutting calories for an active person from 3,000 to 2,500 daily—combined with more exercise could significantly boost the chances (depending on your genes) of making it to age eighty, ninety, or beyond in great health, according to Dr. Roth. Creating a temporary food shortage will also help maintain a desirable weight, which further curbs disease risk and helps extend life.

WHY YOU MUST MOVE

We have always been active. Prior to the development of agriculture, our ancestors were vigorously active for up to twenty hours a week. Our bodies are meant to be fit; when they aren't kept in shape, they break down. On the other hand, fit bodies reap benefits beyond many people's wildest dreams. People in their second fifty years not only can slow the aging process, they might even be able to reverse it with exercise. A weekly routine that mimics our ancient activity levels, with endurance activity such as walking combined with strength training exercise such as lifting weights, helps

- prevent bone deterioration and even reverses bone loss,
- reduce the risk of developing heart disease,
- maintain a desirable weight,
- reduce the risk of losing your independence later in life due to frailty and weakness,
- possibly reduce cancer risk, and
- provide the essential vitality to enjoy those extra years.

In fact, unfit people at any age can reduce their risk of dying prematurely by up to 50 percent by becoming fit, and active people look two decades younger than their couch potato counterparts. See chapter 6 for a detailed description of why our bodies thrive on exercise, why it can turn back the hands of time, and how to do it right.

Stone Age Secret #3: Stay Healthy and Mentally Alert Throughout Life

Staying mentally alert and physically robust is essential to survival. Our ancestors who accomplished this were the ones who lived and reproduced. We are their descendants, and our bodies require the same nutrients, foods, activity levels, and lifestyles to survive with gusto.

To maximize our mental and physical health, we must follow the steps outlined in the Original Dozen on page 38. Our bodies thrive on the whole foods, activity, and relaxation that were part of our evolution for hundreds of thousands of generations. Ignoring these basic needs is like yanking a goldfish out of water and then being surprised when it suffers and dies in the open air. Nurture your body, mind, and being with ancient tender loving care and you will stack your evolutionary deck in favor of living disease free, vitally, and long. As one person who switched to the Origin Diet said, "Being healthy is well worth the effort!"

4

Evolutionary Weight Loss

- If evolution could carefully organize and harmonize 10 trillion cells into the spectacular human body, why didn't it design a shut-off valve for chocolate cravings and out-of-control appetites?
- How can a body so splendidly designed be so flawed as to allow a person to gain hundreds of pounds beyond a reasonable weight?
- If survival of the fittest is the main biological drive, why would our bodies so willingly become unfit?
- Why do we crave the very foods we shouldn't eat?

To answer these questions, you must view the human body from a Stone Age, not a "New" Age, perspective. In the days of woolly mammoths, cave dwellings, and ice ages, fat was beautiful. It was also rare. For millions of years our ancestors cycled between feast and famine. Even during the best of times, their choices were only wild plants and ultra-lean game, and a handful of nuts, seeds, beans, and honey. The skinny ones with high metabolisms died from starvation at the first sign of a drought. Those able to store a little body fat lived to pass their genes to their children, who passed them on to the next generation, and ultimately to us. Our body fat is as fundamental to survival as our will to live.

Why Our Bodies Are Made to Gain Weight

Our bodies may have evolved a complex system to hoard fat, but obesity is virtually nonexistent in the wild. From Paleolithic rock-wall paintings of our ancient ancestors to modern-day hunter-gatherers and everyone who has adopted the Origin Diet in this book, people stay fit when they eat in tune with their evolutionary roots.* They also don't gain weight as they age.

Obesity and middle-age spread are New Age phenomena. Photographs taken in the early 1900s show lumberjacks, railroad workers, farmers, grandparents, and even the wealthy as lean, since only 1 in every 150 people in those days was pudgy. By the 1980s, that number had increased to 1 in 4, by 1994 1 in 3 people was battling the bulge, and according to a recent report from the National Institutes of Health, the numbers have jumped to 55 percent of American adults. Obesity is on the rise in country after country, as each adopts westernized lifestyles.

Don't blame obesity on your genes! "It takes eons for our genes to adapt to changes in our environment," says Tom Baranowski, Ph.D., professor of behavioral nutrition at Baylor College of Medicine in Houston, "while escalating obesity is a phenomenon of the past few decades." Today's habits have resulted in more people being fat and fat people getting fatter. The average American is twenty-six pounds heavier today than one hundred years ago. Baranowski warns us, "There is every reason to believe this trend will get worse unless we make serious changes in our lifestyles." John Foreyt, Ph.D., obesity expert at Baylor College of Medicine, agrees and predicts that at the rate the average waistline is expanding in the United States, everyone will be overweight in another one hundred years or so unless people make conscious efforts to return to more natural diets and exercise levels. In short, genetics might increase a person's susceptibility to obesity, but those ticking genes only explode into a weight problem with the help of habits.

---

*Okay, there are the famous "Venus" statues portraying fat Stone Age females, but these are thought to be products of artistic license, not realistic portrayals.

TIGHT FITTING GENES

A wealth of research puts the kibosh on the belief that out-of-control genes have caused the escalating rates of obesity. For example:

• Skinny hunter-gatherers—from native Americans to Australian Aborigines—who adopt Western lifestyles always gain weight.

• The Tarahumara Indians, who traditionally eat very-low-fat diets, gained an average of 8.5 pounds and their cholesterol levels skyrocketed by 38 percent within five weeks of eating the affluent American diet.

• On the tiny island of Nauru in the Pacific, 70 percent of the women and 65 percent of the men became obese and one in every three people is now diabetic as a result of trading traditional diets of fish and vegetables for potato chips and beer and active lifestyles for lounge chairs.

• Body weight has doubled as Japanese men move from Japan to Hawaii and then to California, adopting higher-fat diets.

• Obesity rates doubled in the past thirty years as Japanese children switched from vegetables, rice, and fish to more Western diets containing animal fat, vegetable oils, and sugar.

• Obesity trends in other countries parallel increased fat and calorie intakes and decreased activity and intake of plants.

• When people return to eating styles more in tune with their evolutionary roots, they lose weight.

THRIFTY GENES

Granted, obesity begets obesity. Children have an 80 percent chance of becoming obese if both parents are obese, a 40 percent chance if one parent is obese, and only a 7 percent chance if both parents are lean. This family tie is a product of "thrifty genes" or a genetically based ability to get and store calories with exceptional efficiency.

Nowhere have thrifty genes been more obvious than with the Pima Indians. Their ancestors who settled in Arizona and adopted Western lifestyles today have the highest obesity and diabetes rates in the world, while Pima Indians who settled in Mexico and who continue to eat fewer calories and burn lots of calories farming are on average fifty-seven pounds lighter and few develop diabetes.

Everyone gains weight when they eat more and move less, but some people gain more and faster than others. "The very genes that helped humans survive and evolve in a world that demanded high energy expenditures and frequent food shortages are now a liability in a world with ample food and little reason to move. It's our environment, not our genes, that is the problem," says Dr. Foreyt.

THE BATTLE AGAINST BIOLOGY

The First Law of Thermodynamics:
   The amount of stored energy equals the difference between energy intake and work.

We evolved as nibblers and gorgers. Obtaining the 3,000-plus calories needed to survive in pre-agricultural times required pounds, not ounces, of food. Unlike koalas, who live almost exclusively on eucalyptus leaves, our nutritional needs are met only by highly varied diets. "Our bodies evolved on large quantities of diverse foods, so it's understandable that people today typically will eat more if given a variety of choices than if they eat monotonous diets," says Barbara Rolls, Ph.D., at Pennsylvania State University in University Park. Dr. Rolls refers to our drive to eat a variety of food as "sensory specific satiety," which simply means that we tire of the same tastes over and over, but give us a selection of tasty choices and we munch much longer. For example, people eat a third more when allowed to choose from a variety of sandwiches than when given only one type of sandwich.

Our bodies were designed to work hard for food. Gathering food required about twenty hours each week of hunting, stalking, digging, picking, and gathering (a 150-pound person expended about 1,363 calories in activity on most days). To counter high-calorie needs with low-calorie supplies, the human body evolved complex systems to defend against weight loss and to maximize weight gain. Foods rich in carbohydrates, fiber, and protein were abundant throughout our evolutionary history, so our bodies had no reason to evolve a system for storing them, but did develop a satiety button to protect us from excess intakes. That explains why today our bodies have the capacity to store only one day's worth of glycogen and small amounts of protein, and why fiber-rich foods fill us up long before they fill us out.

Fat and sugar are a different story. "We humans have a love affair with fat and sugar that dates back to our most ancient roots when these calorie-dense nutrients were in short supply. It is fat, beyond any other nutrient, that gives food the textures, aromas, and tastes that we desire most. Sugar, on the other hand, makes fat taste good," says Adam Drewnowski, Ph.D., professor in the Departments of Epidemiology and Medicine at the University of Washington in Seattle.

And rightfully so. Fat and sugar were scarce hundreds of thousands of years ago; fat supplied at best only about 20 percent of calories from the occasional wild game, nuts, olives, or avocados, and sugar cravings were satisfied with small amounts of seasonal honey and fruit. Fat was a precious source of calories (supplying more than twice the calories per gram of either protein or starch), and our ancient ancestors had no need to develop an appetite shut-off valve for fat. Instead, when they found a tidbit of fatty food or a sweet plum, they ate all they could get and developed an unlimited capacity to store the extra calories.

A LITTLE GOES A LONG WAY

Even a small shift in the balance of calories in versus calories out is enough to tip the scale. For example, a lean person consumes about 900,000 calories in a year. If that person increased calorie intake by only 2 percent (18,000 calories over the year), the person will gain five pounds. The average adult gains twenty pounds between ages twenty-five and fifty-five years, which requires only a 0.3 percent increase in calories.

Consider the following evolutionary pressures to eat sugar and store fat:

• Our sweet-and-creamy cravings are fueled by a stew of at least fifty appetite-control chemicals in the brain, from galanin, serotonin, and neuropeptide Y to the endorphins and the stress hormones, which drive our desire for fat and sweets and make the experience pleasurable by leaving us feeling euphoric or satisfied.

• Fat is not as satiating as protein, fiber, or carbohydrate, so it is easy to passively overconsume this calorie-dense nutrient.

• Fat cravings might be fueled by the need for certain essential fats, such as linoleic acid in vegetables and the omega-3 fatty acids in fish, needed for brain function and the regulation of hormone-like compounds called prostaglandins that affect numerous body processes, such as reducing heart-disease risk.

• Our bodies efficiently store dietary fat, using only 3 percent of its calories to pack it into fat cells, compared to 23 percent of the calories in starch used to convert it to glycogen for storage. Some researchers even theorize that dietary fat has an obesity-promoting effect in people who easily gain weight. (Women are even better fat storers than men. In evolutionary terms, women's bodies were designed to store fat to assure that a pregnancy would succeed and a developing baby would survive a period of famine. A woman's hips, thighs, and derrière are fat-storing machinery.)

• Fat is a hunter's fuel. It is the preferred fuel for endurance activity, which would have been an advantage in the past when our ancestors tracked wild game for hours and even days.

• We absorb as little as 10 percent of iron and 30 percent of calcium in the diet (these minerals were abundant in Paleolithic diets, so there was no need to conserve), but our body efficiently absorbs 95 percent of the fat in our diets, suggesting that fat was a scarce dietary resource.

• Humans are the only species born with fat stores ("baby fat"), which help insulate our hairless bodies, provide a buffer against malnutrition and infection in the first months of life, and prevent disease and death during the vulnerable months of infancy.

But wait. Our bodies might be programmed to *store* fat, but it's obvious we're not meant to *be* fat. Up until recently, humans were lean. Today, people who are fit are the healthiest, at lowest risk for disease, and live the longest. Why would we so easily put on the pounds when doing so increases our risk for disease, pregnancy complications, and psychosocial problems? It goes against the laws of nature to evolve traits that increase our risk for dying. What's going on?

Our Toxic Environment

The battle of the bulge is a natural response to living in what Kelly Brownell, Ph.D., professor of psychology at Yale University, calls a *toxic environment*. "We are exposed to an unprecedented supply of poor-quality food that is widely available, low cost, heavily promoted, and great tasting," says Brownell. We also now eat substantially fewer of the foods on which our bodies thrived for millions of years. "Today we consume only 15 percent of the fiber, but twice the fat, found in pre-agricultural diets," says Dr. George Armelagos. Modern humans are the only free-living species to have ever eaten processed foods. This new way of eating, combined with an abundance of labor-saving devices, has collided head-on with evolution.

THE PARADOX OF PLENTY
Imagine a Monday morning on the savanna 40,000 years ago. A small band of ultra-fit people are organizing their day. Some head off in search of roots, berries, leaves, and other plants. Several prepare for a daylong search for game. All will graze on plants they find along the way and, it is hoped, will return to camp with enough to feed the group that evening. Each will expend 1,000 to 2,000 calories walking, running, stooping, climbing, digging, and chasing food, and will eat four to five pounds of fibrous plants and extra-lean wild game by sundown. Without the conveniences of high-tech outdoor gear or indoor heating, they will expend additional calories just maintaining body temperature. So it went for hundreds of thousands of years, generation after generation.

Fast-forward to the present, where we drive to the supermarket in our temperature-controlled cars to load shopping carts with prepackaged processed foods. Food is everywhere, it's super-tasty and choices are unlimited. Even staunch willpowers are overwhelmed by a food industry that spends billions of dollars to entice us to overeat, taking our two basic appetite drives—a sensitivity to sugar and a love of fat—and

SUPER TASTES, OVEREATING

Taste was a useful sense in ancient times. It wouldn't have taken many generations for our most ancient ancestors to figure out that the ripest fruit tastes the best. Our Paleolithic grandparents probably waited with bated breath all year for the ripe fruits of summer. Transport that cave dweller to a modern-day store loaded with custard-filled doughnuts, gooey cinnamon rolls, chocolate cupcakes, soda pop, and ice cream, and even though these foods would be alien, that cave dweller would probably choose any one of those items over a familiar juicy strawberry. Having evolved over the ages in a world where only lean meat and plants were available, our ancient bodies respond to a highly tasty doughnut or brownie like . . . well, like a kid in a candy shop. It's a natural instinct for what is called "supernormal stimuli."

All animals respond to cues in the environment and will select the cues that are the strongest. For example, a brooding goose instinctively retrieves eggs that roll from her nest. Place a tennis ball nearby and the goose retrieves the ball, not the egg, because to the goose, the ball looks the most egg-like. Supernormal stimuli set off all the senses, especially our taste. Laboratory animals maintain ideal body weights when fed animal chow, but overeat and become obese when fed a wide variety of tasty "people" food. Just like a lab rat, we are more likely to choose banana-cream pie over a banana, a potato chip over a baked potato, or a granola bar over a bowl of plain oatmeal—that is, unless we rein in our appetites.

exploiting them to sell high-calorie, high-fat, high-sugar foods on every street corner. As a result, we eat two to four times more fat, sugar, and salt than any person or animal has ever eaten in the history of the world. "Our energy intake has increased by five hundred calories just since the 1930s, and at least two hundred calories of that has been in the past decade," says John Foreyt.

We have always been a species that liked large portions. It takes a lot of wild greens and roots to fuel a vigorous lifestyle. Our ancestors didn't have calculators to tally calories or fat grams; they depended on the weight of food. Like them, we apparently feel full only when we've eaten a given-weight of food, be it oil-drenched pasta salad or grated zucchini. "People help themselves to a consistent amount of food, regardless of the calories. That's why the energy load of a meal is so important today for weight management," says Dr. Rolls. While our ancestors thrived on pounds of plants, we've cut back to a few four-ounce servings a day, yet are eating unprecedented amounts of calorie-

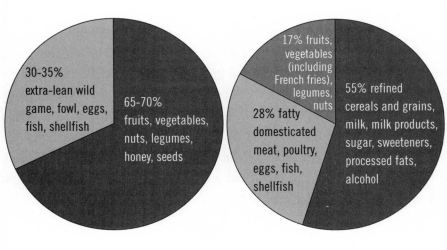

Hunter-Gatherer Diets

30-35% extra-lean wild game, fowl, eggs, fish, shellfish

65-70% fruits, vegetables, nuts, legumes, honey, seeds

Modern Diets

17% fruits, vegetables (including French fries), legumes, nuts

28% fatty domesticated meat, poultry, eggs, fish, shellfish

55% refined cereals and grains, milk, milk products, sugar, sweeteners, processed fats, alcohol

Our bodies evolved on wild plants and game, but today those foods have been replaced with new, processed foods high in fat, sugar, and salt, and low in vitamins, minerals, and fiber.

dense foods. To put it simply: if a pound of food left you feeling full, you could eat a pound of chocolate for 2,330 calories, or munch like a cave dweller on a pound of wild greens that supplies only 100 calories.

Our instinct is to go for large portions, so it's no surprise that we're attracted to today's super-value meals, supersized soda pop, and two-for-one offers. The portions of everything except vegetables keep getting bigger. "Restaurant portions are so big that people can't eat it all. A slice of pie can weigh up to two thirds of a pound!" exclaims Dr. Armelagos. Other examples include:

- A typical muffin or bagel is five times the recommended serving, according to the USDA.
- We gobble 16 cups, not the recommended 3 cups, of movie popcorn during a show.
- Commercial cinnamon rolls supply eight times the calories of traditional servings.
- Soft drinks are served in two-fisted glasses and contain up to 800 calories.

We are the first generation in the entire history of our planet to live with a glut of food without famine. "Our food dilemma is much like the Henry VIII versus Oprah effect," says Dr. Armelagos. "It took up to one hundred people to plant, harvest, prepare, and serve the food needed to feed a fat king, but today it takes personal trainers and private chefs to keep the weight off." The struggle for survival is no longer the effort to find food, but to keep from gobbling too much of the wrong stuff. Yet we skimp on the foods that our bodies need the most.

A CULTURE OF EASE

The new world order is one of minimal movement. Even a century ago, no one exercised; daily life was strenuous enough. Energy expenditure has dropped a staggering 60 percent just since the late twentieth century! Now less than one in ten people is active for more than thirty min-

EATING OUT IS DOING US IN

We are eating out more than ever before, with forty cents of every food dollar spent at restaurants. A typical meal at even an ordinary restaurant tops the charts at 1,000 calories, and that's without appetizers and dessert! Why do we eat so much when we eat out, and how can we cut back?

PROBLEM #1: Restaurant food, especially fast-food fare, is high in fat, salt, and sugar.

Solution: Choose salads, steamed vegetables, grilled meats, and other low-calorie options.

PROBLEM #2: Portions are enormous and we have a tendency to clean our plates.

Solution: Split entrées with a friend or order à la carte.

PROBLEM #3: People eat more when they eat with others, which again would date back to prehistory when you were motivated to get your share when someone brought food into camp. The more drawn out the meal, the more we eat.

Solution: Eat a healthful snack to curb hunger before eating out. Sip on water, rather than eat another chip or appetizer, at the restaurant. Ask for a doggie bag and bag half the entrée before you begin eating.

PROBLEM #4: We are more apt to have a glass of wine or other alcoholic beverage when "treating" ourselves to a restaurant meal. You definitely need a plan regarding alcohol. "Alcohol disinhibits a person so that once you start drinking you are likely to eat more," says Thomas Wadden, Ph.D., professor of psychology and the director of the Weight and Eating Disorders Program at the University of Pennsylvania. Even one light beer or one wine spritzer can topple your willpower.

Solution: Don't order alcoholic beverages when eating out, or drink two glasses of water for every alcoholic beverage.

utes a day. We opt for garage door openers, remote controls, computers, electric can openers, riding lawn mowers, and spectator sports. When given the choice between stairs or escalators, most will wait in line for the escalator, while the stairs sit empty. Developers omit sidewalks from their planned communities, while gasoline sales and hours of television viewing parallel the escalating obesity rate. "We don't walk anymore, can speed dial to order pizza, and our cars are designed with cup holders. Now there are even plug-in microwaves in cars," says Dr. Drewnowski. As Dr. Foreyt says, "With leisure time spent in sedentary pursuits and work usually done sitting, our lifestyles have overwhelmed our genes." We now live in an environment opposite from the one that shaped our evolution—the drive to conserve energy has been replaced by the need to expend much more of it.

Our land of plenty also explains why childhood obesity is on the rise. Gone are the days when kids walked to school, played hide and seek for hours, and rode their bikes until sundown. Like adults, our children sit. They watch three or more hours of television a day, which equates to a minimum of 16,425 hours (almost two years) of TV viewing between the ages of two and seventeen years. That's not counting the time spent sitting in front of a computer, Nintendo, or video game, all of which rev metabolism no more than a nap. "The strongest predictor of childhood obesity is hours spent in front of a television or computer screen," warns Dr. Foreyt. The problem mounts with age as children become less active as they grow up.

Working Against Your Fat Genes

We tackle the weight issue with fad diets and diet pills, but these are as effective for managing weight as a mythical drug to repair the damage caused by smoking. Granted, weight is temporarily lost on fad diets, but 95 percent of it is gained back, and more. That's because you're not playing on an even field. Withholding food from your body is as unnatural as holding your breath. There are at least thirty mechanisms in the body designed over millions of years to fend off weight loss and encourage weight gain. Any attempt or threat to limit fuel is interpreted as an Ice Age food shortage, triggering the body's natural defenses against weight loss:

- Severely cut calories, skip meals, or eat erratically and metabolism slows to preserve energy. "People skip meals in an effort to save calories, which only backfires and inevitably increases cravings, lowers resistance to food temptations later in the day, and usually leads to overeating," says C. Wayne Callaway, M.D., at George Washington University in Washington, D.C.
- Restrict carbohydrates and a symphony of appetite-control chemicals in the brain triggers uncontrollable urges to binge on sweets. "Appetite-regulating chemicals are upset when people go on quick-weight-loss diets, which can lead to overeating," says Sarah Leibowitz, Ph.D., at Rockefeller University in New York City.
- Deprivation leads to obsession. Tell yourself you can't have certain foods and those are the foods you will crave the most.
- Cut out entire categories of food and you'll crave variety. "Most fad diets work in the short term because they limit choices and people will eat less on monotonous diets, even if all they eat is doughnuts. But our instinct is to eat a variety of foods, and eventually the pendulum will swing from abstinence to overeating when we slip off the diet," says Dr. Rolls. Evolutionary-wise, your body is stocking up before the next diet begins.

DRINKS AND DIET FOODS

Soda pop sales have skyrocketed since the 1970s, right along with waist-lines. Could there be a connection? Possibly. Your appetite controls don't compensate for the calories consumed in beverages (why should they when calorie-free water was the only beverage your ancient ances-tors drank?). Consequently, you eat the same food plus the extra calories in the beverage. Drink a thirty-two-ounce cola every day and you'll be three pounds heavier by the end of the month. Drink a glass of wine with your dinner every night and you'll be a pound heavier after a month.

The Diet Paradox

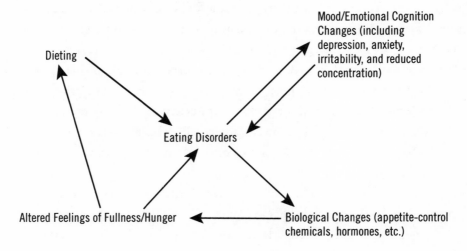

Severe calorie restriction triggers the body's natural defenses against weight loss, usually resulting in overeating, disturbed signals of satiety and hunger, and mood changes.

Diet foods also don't work. Tell us we're eating fat free, and we eat more. In a study conducted by Dr. Rolls, women ate more for lunch when they thought they were snacking on low-fat yogurt than they did when they were told the yogurt was full fat, regardless of the actual fat and calorie contents. This mind-over-calories phenomenon might explain why obesity rates continue to rise despite increasing use of fake sugars (it's too soon to tell if fake fats will help us cut back on calories, but my guess is they won't).

OUTSMARTING YOUR FAT GENES

While fad diets and diet soft drinks don't work, cutting calories without sacrificing nutrition is one way to work with your body's natural weight balance. "Calorie restriction is the only manipulation known to improve both average and maximal lifespan," says Dr. George Roth.

The secret is reducing calories, while still feeling satisfied and staying healthy. That means cutting back on unnecessary "modern" calories from fat, sugar, and alcohol, while leaving every bite chock-full of the foods on which we evolved—fruits, vegetables, whole grains, legumes, fish, and other minimally processed food, plus nonfat milk products to ensure calcium intake. Even a modest reduction—say cutting calories for an active person from 2,500 to 2,000 daily (or maintaining calories and increasing energy expenditure by this amount)—could significantly boost the chances of living long, healthfully, and lean, according to Dr. Roth. Following that advice is easier than you might think. Just read on.

Stone Age Secrets #1 and #2: How to Eat Pounds of Food and Lose Weight

"The Origin Diet is so easy. No gimmicks and all the food is readily available, even if a person doesn't cook."—Kathy

"After only a week or two on this eating plan, I noticed I had more energy, felt in control of my cravings, and my pants were looser!"—Nicki

"I felt lighter, fresher, healthier within one week of starting the Origin Diet."—Tim

"I wasn't even trying to lose weight and still dropped a pound a week on this eating plan."—Rollie

"I'm eating more often and much healthier than I have in the past and I'm still losing weight."—Emma

Your body was designed to be lean and fit. Embracing the Stone Age Secrets #1 (Stay strong and lean) and #2 (Focus on wild or natural foods) will help you return to a diet and activity level more in tune with your origins. In fact, return to our original way of eating and your body will respond as if it were coming home from a long, exhausting trip. This is the best way to work with your basic instincts and to stay fit for life. Granted, in today's world of unlimited food and energy-conserving conveniences, it might be difficult for some people to attain this fitness level, but everyone can be healthy, lose excess fat weight, and more closely approach the body they were meant to have.

Despite the seemingly overwhelming biology that fuels our drive to eat, we have an even more remarkable trait—adaptability. More than any other species on earth, humans are curious, flexible, and quick learners. Our eating habits are as much learned as they are innate, which is one of the reasons our species survived when others, like the Neanderthals, didn't. Since our current eating habits are entirely learned, they can be replaced by reawakening our original habits. This has been proven time and time again when people adopt the Origin Diet. As Dolores said, "I feel satisfied and find myself turning to healthy foods when a craving hits, rather than cookies and cheese like in the past." The secret is to make the adjustment gradually, avoid feeling deprived, and follow the guidelines below.

Mother Nature's Seven Basic Weight-Management Guidelines

GUIDELINE 1:
Accept that managing your weight is a lifelong process, not a short-term problem. You must customize the Origin eating program in chapter 5 to permanently fit your life. Remember, you want to both maximize your health and trim your waistline. Think of your weight as a marriage, something that takes daily commitment, attention, focus, patience, and love.

GUIDELINE 2:
Follow the activity guidelines outlined in chapter 6. "Daily physical activity shifts the body from energy excess to energy need, so what is considered overeating when you're sedentary is fueling your body when you're fit," says Dr. Drewnowski.

GUIDELINE 3:
Fill up on Mother Nature's diet foods. It is the weight of food, not its calories, that fills you up. A low-calorie meal will satisfy you as much as

a high-calorie meal, as long as they weigh the same. So work with this instinct by loading the plate with foods that weigh lots, but have few calories. That means watery and fiber-rich fruits, vegetables, whole grains, and legumes. Both take up more room in your stomach than processed foods, so you feel full on fewer calories. Pile more vegetables and less cheese on your pizza, add more vegetables and less fatty meat to stir fries, and dilute the calories in a brown bag lunch by adding more fruit and less potato salad.

Calories: A Weight Issue

It's the weight of food, not its calories, that satisfies our hunger pangs. The secret is to eat foods that weigh a lot, but pack few calories. That means focusing on foods with high water and fiber contents. Here's a list of the best and the worst when it comes to weighty calories.

SOME OF THE BEST (LOW ENERGY DENSITY)	CALORIES PER OUNCE
Cooked spinach or chard, raw bell pepper	7
Strawberries	8
Cooked broccoli, grapefruit	9
Melon, nonfat milk	10
Raw carrot	12
Soft tofu	17
Steamed shrimp	28

SOME OF THE WORST (HIGH ENERGY DENSITY)	
Hamburger	83
Ice cream	90
Marshmallows	100
Rice cakes	105
Buttered popcorn	140
Potato chips	152

Here are three reasons why natural fiber-rich foods are the best way to lose weight and keep it off:

1. Our bodies evolved on fiber-rich foods, which take more time to chew, so our brains have more time to process information from the stomach that we've had enough—before we eat too much.
2. Fiber-rich foods are naturally low in fat and calories, so you can eat more food for fewer calories. Kathy, who lost weight following the Origin Diet, said, "For the first time in years, I'm satisfied after a meal. Food has more flavor. The best part is that I can eat all I want."
3. According to a U.S. Department of Agriculture study, fiber reduces the number of calories you absorb, reducing women's intake by about 90 calories and men's by about 130 calories a day. Over the course of a year, that could mean losing 9 to 13½ pounds!

Design your weight-management plan around the following original habits:

• Eat two fruits and/or vegetables at every meal and snack. People who have followed this one guideline in the Origin Diet have lost up to thirty pounds in fourteen weeks. Richard commented, "I snack on fruits and vegetables throughout the day and don't seem to eat as much food to feel full on this diet, which probably explains why I've lost eight pounds in the last five weeks and never felt deprived!"
• Snack on beans. Bean spreads, such as black bean dip or hummus made without tahini, are especially filling, since they are high in fiber and water, but low in fat.
• Serve soup. "Broth-based soups are satisfying foods because they tend to be low in fat and high in fiber and water, the two ingredients that add volume without adding calories," says Dr. Rolls. Start meals with a bowl of tomato or vegetable soup and you'll eat less of the remaining courses than if you had the fried potato skins for an appetizer. Or make a meal out of soup. (See the recipe section at the end of the book for several delicious soups.)

- Emphasize variety. Our species thrives on variety. Overeating a variety of fruit, vegetables, and even nonfat dairy foods does not put on the pounds. Let this instinct work in your favor by stocking your refrigerator, kitchen cabinets, and desk drawer at work with a variety of wholesome, low-fat foods, including cut-up fresh fruit with yogurt dip, baby carrots, whole grain crackers with soy or nonfat cheese, or bean dips with whole wheat pita bread.

- Drink water. Mother Nature's diet drink, water has no calories, yet fills you up. Sip water just before or while eating to add weight to the meal.

HOW VARIED IS YOUR DIET?

Variety is the key to a healthful diet, but only if you eat a variety of the right foods. How many of the following foods do you eat on any four days? If you check at least twenty-seven, your diet is probably varied and healthy. If you check less than seventeen, you should consider expanding your nutritional horizons.

1. Dark green vegetables (spinach, chard, kale, etc.)
2. Citrus fruit
3. Orange or yellow vegetables
4. Tomatoes and tomato products
5. Starchy vegetables, not fried (sweet potatoes, yams, etc.)
6. Cruciferous vegetables (cabbage, broccoli, cauliflower, asparagus, Brussels sprouts, etc.)
7. Leaf lettuce
8. Berries
9. Melons
10. Other colorful vegetables
11. Other colorful fruits
12. Other pale-colored vegetables and fruits (white potatoes, jicama, parsnips, radishes, iceberg lettuce, bananas, etc.)

13. Fruit juice
14. Vegetable juice
15. Whole wheat bread, bagels, crackers, tortillas, etc.
16. Other whole grains (brown rice, oats, pasta, cornmeal, quinoa, barley, etc.)
17. Whole grain cereals (Shredded Wheat, Nutri-Grain, Grape-Nuts, etc.)
18. Nonfat or 1 percent low-fat milk
19. Nonfat or 1 percent low-fat plain yogurt
20. Nonfat or low-fat cheese or soy cheese
21. Eggs
22. Chicken or turkey breast meat, skinless
23. Fish
24. Shellfish
25. Cooked dried beans and peas (beans, lentils, split peas, etc.)
26. Soybean products (tofu, soymilk, textured vegetable protein, tempeh, miso)
27. Nuts and nut butters, soy butter
28. Seeds
29. Olive oil, canola oil
30. Honey
31. Water
32. Salty snacks, convenience foods, fast foods, processed foods
33. Sweet baked items, desserts, ice cream, and other foods containing sugar
34. Red meat, pork, dark poultry meat, full-fat sour cream or cream cheese, margarine, butter, and oils
35. Refined breads, cereals, and grains (white bread, white rice, white flour tortillas, etc.)
36. Candy, soft drinks, and sugar

GUIDELINE 4:

Listen to your body. Don't use food as a tranquilizer when anxious, a mood elevator when depressed, a comforter when lonely, an entertainer when bored, or a lover when emotionally starved. "Talk through, rather than eat through, feelings," recommends Dr. Thomas Wadden. Ask yourself before you eat, "What am I feeling?" Eat only if you are physically hungry. Fulfill your emotional needs by means other than foods, such as daily exercise, spending time in nature, developing close friendships, meditating, or even counseling. (See chapter 7.)

The good news is that when you turn to healthy foods in the Origin Diet, you feel satisfied and are less likely to overeat in response to emotions. Susan went on the Origin Diet and commented, "I've always been a stress eater. When I was tired, I'd turn to food as a treat to pick me up. But now I don't go looking for treats anymore, I don't even have the desire to wander into the kitchen looking for a snack. Best of all, I feel great."

SNACKS FOR ALL SEASONS

The following twenty-eight snacks supply approximately 100 calories and help fill you up without filling you out:

- 10-ounce glass of vanilla soymilk (93.6 calories)
- 6 ounces nonfat plain yogurt (94 calories)
- ¾ cup nonfat milk warmed and mixed with 1 packet sugar-free cocoa mix (112 calories)
- 1 cup fresh-squeezed orange juice (111 calories)
- Garbanzo Cilantro Dip* (96 calories)
- 1½ cups fresh blueberries (102 calories)
- 2 cups cantaloupe cubes, drizzled with lime juice (112 calories)
- 2½ cups fresh strawberries (108 calories)
- 1 banana, sliced and sprinkled with nutmeg (104 calories)
- 1 slice whole wheat toast with 1 teaspoon apricot preserves (98.4 calories)
- ½ whole wheat bagel (small) with 1 teaspoon fat-free cream cheese (102 calories)

*See recipe on page 249.

- 2 cups fresh spinach sautéed in 1 teaspoon olive oil with 2 minced garlic cloves (102 calories)
- 1 medium sweet potato, sliced into strips and baked until crispy (117 calories)
- 2 cups asparagus sautéed in 2 teaspoons soy sauce and 2 tablespoons chicken broth (97.6 calories)
- 2 cups tossed salad greens with 1 medium sliced tomato, 2 tablespoons kidney beans, and 1 tablespoon oil-free dressing (107 calories)
- ½ cup steamed corn kernels mixed with ⅓ cup chopped sweet red peppers (101 calories)
- 1 slice whole wheat French bread (96 calories)
- 3½ cups air-popped popcorn (107 calories)
- 1 cup mango slices (107 calories)
- 1 tablespoon crunchy peanut butter (94 calories)
- 3½ cups slightly steamed yellow zucchini, cut into rounds and salted (101 calories)
- 26 baby carrots (98.8 calories)
- 1 cup tomato soup made with ¼ cup nonfat milk and ½ cup water (111 calories)
- 2 ounces water-packed tuna, drained and mixed with 2 teaspoons fat-free mayonnaise, and served on 2 whole wheat crackers (98.8 calories)
- 1 cup shredded cabbage and 1 ounce firm-cubed tofu sautéed in 2 teaspoons peanut sauce (just until warmed, 2 minutes). Top with 2 tablespoons chopped cilantro (105 calories)
- ¼ whole wheat pita dipped in ⅓ cup fat-free refried beans with 1 teaspoon salsa (105 calories)
- 1 tablespoon orange juice concentrate, ½ banana, and 2 apricot halves blended to make a smoothie (97.2 calories)
- ½ cup cooked brown rice mixed with 3 tablespoons cooked black beans, seasoned with cumin, salt, and pepper to taste (96.6 calories)

GUIDELINE 5:

Adopt any or all of the following suggestions, which help you work with, rather than against, your drive to feel comfortably full on fewer calories. The more tips you follow, the greater the benefits.

- *Eat small meals and snacks.* Large meals stretch the stomach's capacity, so you need more food to feel full. Cut back and your stomach's capacity also shrinks, so you feel full on less. Pare down your portions and you might feel a little more hungry for the first few weeks, but before long you'll notice your appetite and hunger have restabilized at a lower intake. "It makes sense that the body is better adapted to small doses of fuel and nutrients all day long than trying to handle a glut of food every so often," says Sharon Edelstein, research scientist at George Washington University in Washington, D.C., and lead researcher on a study that linked snacking with a lower risk for disease. Our ancient ancestors evolved by grazing—not gorging—on nuts, berries, roots, and small game. Feasts were rare and probably occurred only when someone in the tribe slew a woolly mammoth or other large animal. In short, our bodies were designed for nibbling on high-fiber, low-fat foods, not the "gorge 'n' fast" eating style of modern society. Eating regularly prevents feeling famished, which can lead to overeating. Linda, who lost eight pounds in six weeks on the Origin Diet, said, "I used to be famished when I sat down at mealtime, but now I'm just comfortably hungry and tend to eat less as a result."
- *Limit alcohol.* One to two drinks a week is fine, but any more and you're adding extra calories that add pounds without helping you feel full. You also eat more when you're drinking. Calories in alcohol can't be stored, so they're used for energy, allowing more fat from a meal to be stored.
- *Eat slowly.* It takes a while for messages from the stomach to reach the brain. If you eat quickly, you will consume more calories before the brain realizes you're full.
- *Try nuts.* One of the few natural sources of fat and a good source of protein and fiber, nuts are surprisingly satisfying. A study from Purdue

University found that people who ate nuts compensated for the calories by cutting back elsewhere. But don't go overboard, since nuts are high-calorie foods.

• *Make it tasty.* Flavor is critical to our appetites. "Flavor is so important to us that primitive people would trade scarce food for an unusual spice, even if the flavor was foreign to them," says Dr. Rolls. See the box below for ideas on how to make food flavorful without adding calories.

TWENTY WAYS TO MAKE FOOD TASTY WITHOUT CALORIES

Taste needn't rely on fat and sugar. As the recipes in this book show, you can make food deliciously flavorful by adding a number of low-calorie ingredients, such as any of the following:

1. Canned chiles: Add whole chiles to a grilled chicken sandwich or diced chiles to soups, scrambled eggs, pita sandwiches, or sprinkle on tortillas.
2. Dried cranberries. Great in marinades for baked chicken. Add to quick breads, spinach salads, chicken salads, and rice dishes.
3. Portobello mushrooms: Marinate and grill like hamburger, slice grilled and add to salads or pasta dishes, or use instead of meat for sandwiches.
4. Canned roasted red or yellow peppers: Add to a grilled cheese sandwich, blend them with some cayenne and drizzle over a creamed vegetable soup, egg dishes, pasta sauces (cold and hot), or add as a topping with cheese for crackers.
5. Fresh cilantro: Add to fruit- or tomato-based salsa to accompany fish or poultry. Add to curried chicken salads with celery, apples, and grapes. Add to a bean burrito, fruit or vegetable salads, vinaigrette dressings, black beans, or rice dishes.
6. Red onions: Slice thin and add to salads, sandwiches, bean dips, or egg dishes.

7. Honey: Drizzle over yogurt, warm brown rice with pistachios, or sliced apples. Sweeten mashed sweet potatoes with honey. Mix with mustard, orange juice, balsamic vinegar, and herbs as a marinade for chicken.

8. Fresh parsley: Mix with lemon and pepper and drizzle over grilled fish. Mix with minced garlic and whole wheat bread crumbs or wheat germ for a savory crust for potato dishes or chicken. Mix with olive oil and garlic for a pesto sauce for mashed potatoes.

9. Mint: Add to chopped tomatoes and cucumbers, rice dishes, and beans.

10. Sundried tomatoes: Use in pasta salads, sandwich spreads, vegetable dips, or as an extra topping on pizza. Mix into sautéed zucchini or as an accompaniment to grilled eggplant. Blend with olives, garlic, and balsamic vinegar to make a spicy spread for grilled vegetable sandwiches.

11. Fresh ginger: Combine with curry to flavor chicken, add to hot or iced tea, use to season steamed vegetables such as pea pods or carrots. Use as a topping along with green onions on roasted fish. Add to stir fries, tofu dishes, or salad dressings.

12. Horseradish: Use in potato dishes, vegetable dips with dill, vegetable or chicken wraps with fat-free sour cream, spicy soup like gumbo, turkey burgers (ginger is good here, too), cold potato salad, or cold green beans.

13. Lemon: Add grated rind (called zest) to fruit salads. The juice can put a tangy taste in couscous, gazpacho, and dressings, and can be used as marinade for fish.

14. Fresh herbs: Fresh always tastes better than dried. Add fresh basil to pasta, tomatoes or other vegetables, bread dough, or even mango slices (basil and lemon are a good match). Fresh rosemary accents any meat, as well as pasta dishes, roasted vegetables, lima beans, peas, or squash. Fresh dill is an excellent flavor for fish, chicken, omelets and other egg dishes, salads, beets, cabbage, potatoes, or cucumbers. Fresh oregano is excellent in Italian, Greek, or Mexican dishes.

15. Hoisin sauce: Use as a glaze with garlic, cilantro, and ginger for chicken. Add to steamed green beans.
16. Pine nuts: Add a few to stuffings, pesto sauce, pilafs, and fillings for poultry or vegetables, such as eggplant or large zucchini.
17. Crushed red pepper flakes or Tabasco: Sprinkle on pizza, pasta dishes, salads, or soups. Add to olive oil or sour cream dips, rice dishes, or bean salads. Mix into cornbread batter or bread dough.
18. Tamarind: Add to mixed steamed vegetables, fresh orange juice, salad dressing, and sauces for fish.
19. Salsa: Make your own by experimenting with grilled corn, vine-ripened tomatoes, garlic, red onions, and chiles. Or try fruit salsa made from mango, jicama, and black beans. Try adding rice wine vinegar, fresh mint, lime juice, fresh herbs, avocado, or cilantro.
20. Sherry: Add a tablespoon to soups, sauces, marinades, or fruit glazes.

GUIDELINE 6:

Add a one-day fast to your routine. Your ancient ancestors sometimes went without. Create a temporary food shortage by just saying "no" to food every so often. Drink only fruit juices, tea, and other mild beverages for one day once or twice a month. You will be surprised what you'll learn about your relationship to food when you avoid it for a day!

GUIDELINE 7:

Keep a food journal. Our Stone Age relatives didn't need to keep track, but today monitoring what you eat, how much, and when is a tried-and-true habit of successful weight managers. Make sure to accurately record serving sizes (people typically underestimate how much they eat and overestimate how much they exercise).

Most important, follow the guidelines in chapter 5 for how to eat and in chapter 6 for how to exercise. I promise, if you adopt these suggestions, you will lose weight and feel the best you've ever felt!

PART II

■ ■ ■

Re-creating a Lifestyle

5

The Origin Diet

"There is something about the mind-set of being on the Origin Diet. It's such a positive focus—what you can have, rather than what you can't have. It also helps that there are no complicated formulas, just common sense and healthy eating." —Susan

"This way of eating gets easier the longer you stick with it. And the payoffs are worth it! I have more energy, sleep better, my cravings have stopped, and I seem to handle stress better." —Linda

"What a refreshing switch from all the diet hype these days! I feel great, lost weight, and want to stick with this for life."—Katherine

It's no surprise that people who adopt the Origin Diet repeatedly say they feel better. Our bodies were fine-tuned over millions of years—growing increasingly stronger, taller, and smarter—by eating foods native to the environment. Fueling your body with the foods on which it thrives *should* give you a new lease on life!

Granted, times have changed. The mammoths, mastodons, and saber-toothed tigers are gone; most of our fruits and vegetables are cultivated, not wild; and fresh water now comes bottled. Despite all that, we can return to ancient eating styles and still live in today's world. Better yet, it's much easier than you might think.

(123)

BASIC GUIDELINES FOR THE ORIGIN DIET

- Eat regularly, starting with breakfast and every four to five hours throughout the day.
- Keep meals and snacks light.
- Eat slowly and until comfortably full, not stuffed.
- Never allow yourself to become ravenous. Always eat when comfortably hungry and before feeling starved.
- Include at least two fruits and/or vegetables at every meal and at least one at every snack for a minimum of eight a day. More is better.
- Include two to three servings of calcium-rich foods—such as 1 cup nonfat milk, nonfat yogurt, or calcium-fortified soymilk, or 4 ounces canned salmon with bones—in your daily diet.
- Include at least three servings of starchy vegetables—such as sweet potato, yams, white potato, winter squash, or corn—in your daily diet.
- Include at least six servings of whole grains in your daily diet.
- Include at least two servings of low-saturated-fat, protein/iron-rich foods—such as turkey or chicken breast, fish and shellfish, cooked dried beans and peas, tofu and soy products—each day.
- If you also want to lose weight, cut back slightly on grains and/or fats from olive oil, nuts, and avocados. (See chapter 4.)

Our bodies don't know or care whether needed protein comes from a mastodon or a salmon. Calcium for strong bones can come from two pounds of wild greens or from three glasses of nonfat milk. Vitamin C for healthy eyesight, strong arteries, and vital immune systems can come as easily from a kiwi as a handful of thimbleberry shoots. Each one of the trillions of cells in your body only cares that you consume the same range and amounts of the forty-plus essential nutrients and a wide variety of the thousands of phytochemicals on which those cells and our bodies evolved. You easily can eat according to your evolutionary roots by selecting chin-dribbling strawberries and other fruits, crunchy carrots and other vegetables, and comfort foods like roast chicken and potatoes, and by switching from white to whole wheat bread, from whole milk to nonfat milk, and from sugar to honey. The box on page 124 outlines the basic guidelines. How to put those guidelines into practice is explained in this chapter.

It's an Eating Style, Not a Diet

Let's get one thing straight before we begin. No one nutrient is an island. No one diet has all the answers. No one food lowers weight or prevents disease. Nuts alone won't save your heart. Grapefruit won't trim your waistline, just as carbohydrates don't make you fat. Beef by itself isn't a killer food. Oat bran is not the answer to diabetes. Vitamin E alone won't boost your immune system. Fish oil capsules by themselves won't solve your mood problems. Even wheat germ isn't a perfect food.

The Origin Diet isn't your typical diet. It doesn't promote one food or a group of foods. It's an eating style, a pattern of fueling your body that reflects your dietary heritage. The closer you follow it, the more you will live in tune with your natural health. The sooner you start, the better, but it's never too late to reap the rewards.

The Origin Pyramid

The Origin Pyramid on page 126 gives you a picture of what the Origin's plate and your food choices should look like. It's slightly different from today's USDA Food Guide Pyramid. Grains, fruits, and vegetables are still the mainstays, but the grains are whole grain only, and they share space with starchy vegetables such as sweet potatoes and corn. Fruits and vegetables are predominant, taking up two layers, one for cooked or dried, and one for raw. Meat and legumes are a modest contributor to the diet; the meat is only extra lean, and the beans are important enough to have their own box. Milk also is important, but it must be primarily nonfat, while the final tier of the Origin Pyramid is taken up by small amounts of honey, eggs, and naturally high fat items like olives, nuts, and

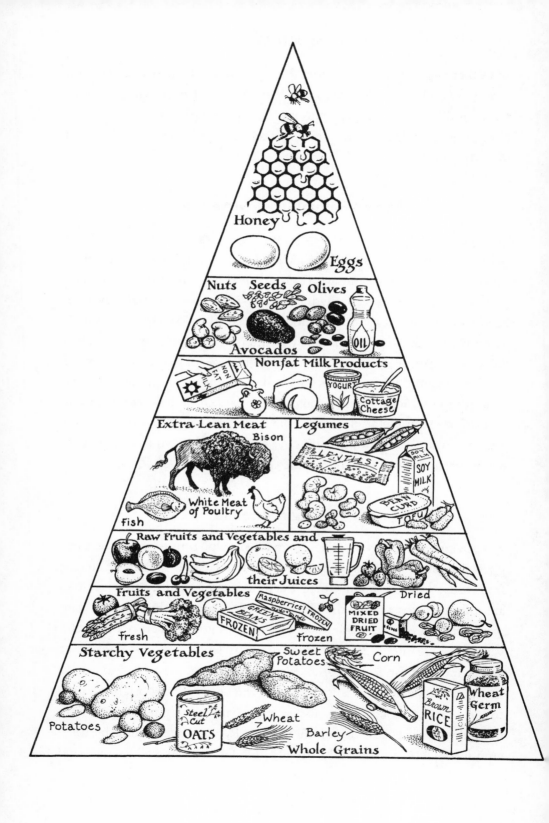

avocados. What you won't find on this pyramid are highly processed foods. Basically, you're designing your menus around foods that you would find in the wild. If it doesn't grow on a tree, bush, vine, or plant; can't be dug up or harvested; isn't hunted; or can't be found in nature, then it probably doesn't belong on your plate.

Back to Basics: The Steps to Evolutionary Eating

The rules for switching from a westernized diet to the Origin Diet are simple and straightforward. Nine of the Twelve original dozen evolutionary steps focus on what and how to eat. (Steps 10 and 11 will be discussed in chapter 6, Step 12 in chapter 7.) They include:

Step 1. Consume eight to ten servings of rainbow-colored fruits and vegetables every day, or at least two at every meal and one at each snack. Some should be raw and some cooked. This is one of the most important tips and should be at the top of your priority list.

Step 2. Carbohydrates are the mainstay of the diet. However, you'll need to make a slight tweak in your daily habits to switch from refined grains and French fries to minimally processed starchy vegetables, whole grains, fruits, legumes, and honey. As a result, your fiber intake will increase to about 35 to 50 grams or more a day. (Hint: When adding fiber to your diet, go slow. Increasing your fiber intake too quickly can result in intestinal gas.)

Step 3. Your protein and iron-rich foods are skinless poultry breast, fish, shellfish, wild game, and legumes. Choose only fat-free milk products. This will reduce saturated fats to about 6 percent of total calories, which is in tune with our original diets.

Step 4. Boost your intake of natural fats, such as the omega-3 fatty acids in fish and flaxseed meal, and the unsaturated fats in nuts, avocados, olives, and olive and canola oils.

Step 5. Graze, don't gorge, by consuming five to six mini-meals throughout the day.

Step 6. Avoid processed foods high in sugar, refined flours, salt, and additives.

Step 7. Drink at least eight glasses of water a day.

Step 8. If your weight creeps up by five pounds or more, voluntarily do what your ancestors were forced to do: create a temporary food shortage by lowering calorie intake and increasing daily activity.

Step 9. Use nutritional supplements responsibly.

Some people who have adopted the Origin Diet found it easy, since they needed only to fine-tune already healthy eating styles. Other people found the process a bit daunting at first, until they realized they didn't need to make all the changes at once. Granted, the more steps you include in your diet, the greater the health benefits, but adding any step to your routine will improve your health. So don't beat yourself up if you don't follow the Origin Diet perfectly. Give yourself credit for small steps toward a healthier eating style. Also, be creative and flexible when incorporating the Origin Diet into your lifestyle. Emma found that she was most motivated to stick with it over the long term if she followed the guidelines during the week, but relaxed the rules on the weekends. Rollie settled into a pattern of following the diet when he was home, and sticking with it about 75 percent of the time when he traveled. The cravings for steak never subsided for Tim, so to stick with the healthier eating plan he included a serving or two each week of red meat. Dolores had no trouble following this eating plan, except that she missed her beloved fig bars, so she planned them into her weekly menus. Natalie decided to keep chocolate in her weekly plan, even though the cravings had stopped. The most important goal is to stick with this healthy eating plan for life; if that means including a few processed foods into your daily or weekly plan, then by all means do it!

It helps to make changes gradually, taking two months to a year to switch from your current eating style to the Origin Diet. The added benefit of making gradual changes is that this allows the body time to adapt. For example, Dr. William Connor found that switching too quickly from a typical high-fat diet to a high-carbohydrate diet can cause a temporary rise in blood triglyceride levels. "You can prevent this rise by eating whole grains and gradually increasing starches and fruits and reducing fat over two to three months." says Dr. Connor.

Here are some of the gradual changes people made as they adopted the Origin Diet:

- Switch from whole milk to 2 percent low-fat, then to 1 percent low-fat, and finally to nonfat milk.
- Use sharp cheddar cheese, rather than mild. You'll use less. Gradually, switch to low-fat cheeses, then to soy cheese.
- Include one extra vegetable serving a day. Increase serving number and size over several months.
- Cut back on your serving size of red meat. Later, cut back on frequency, and finally replace red meat with more beans, chicken breast, and fish.
- If you can't get used to whole grain pasta, then keep your regular pasta and focus on whole grain breads, crackers, and cereals. Use phyllo dough for pie crusts; it isn't whole wheat, but it's low in fat.

Prioritize what steps you will take first. Some changes will have a greater impact on your health than others, so select goals that maximize the benefits from the Origin Diet.

Top priority: These three Origin goals will give you the greatest health benefit for your effort:

- Cut back on saturated fat by eliminating red meat and fatty milk products.
- Boost your intake of omega-3 fats by including several servings weekly of fish in the diet, or by taking fish oil supplements or eating omega-3 fortified foods.
- Include no less than eight, and preferably ten, servings of fruits and vegetables in your daily diet.

Second priority: These two Origin goals will give you an extra health boost. Attempt these once you have successfully accomplished the above three goals:

- Increase fiber by choosing only whole grains.
- Increase your intake of cooked dried beans and peas, lentils, and soy.

Third priority: The following three Origin goals are important considerations after the above five goals have been successfully accomplished:

- Include three servings of nonfat milk or calcium- and vitamin-D-fortified soymilk in the daily diet.
- Supplement responsibly.
- Cut back on salt.

Prioritize your current eating habits. If you can't imagine life without cheese or an occasional bowl of ice cream, then by all means keep these foods in your weekly eating plan. On the other hand, if it doesn't matter whether you eat white or whole wheat bread or drink whole or 1 percent milk, then make these relatively painless substitutions first. Remember, you don't need to follow the diet perfectly. However, the closer you do, the more health rewards you'll reap.

Now let's see how to put those priorities into action!

EVOLUTIONARY DIET QUICK TRICKS

Need a little coaching when it comes to devolving back to your ancestral roots? Here are some easy ways to eat more like your lean 'n' fit ancestors:

- Eat at least two servings daily of dark green vegetables, such as spinach, romaine lettuce, beet greens, collards, or chard. (Add greens to lasagna, casseroles, soups, and stews.)

- Include at least two vitamin-C-rich selections, such as citrus, strawberries, or green pepper daily. (Add orange and grapefruit sections to salads, rice, or grain dishes.)
- Several times a week, pick something from the cabbage family, such as Brussels sprouts, kohlrabi, asparagus, cabbage, broccoli, or cauliflower.
- Add leftover vegetables from last night's dinner to lunchtime soups and salads or add frozen vegetables to canned soups.
- For shish-kabob, skewer more vegetables (including carrots, eggplant, cherry tomatoes, zucchini, onions, potato, or mushrooms) than chicken or fish.
- Experiment with new whole grains: Choose breads that promise 100 percent whole grain on the label, instant brown rice, whole wheat couscous, quinoa, roasted buckwheat groats, barley, amaranth, bulgur, wild rice, and millet.
- When reading labels, choose foods that contain more calories from protein than from fat.
- When choosing canned goods, purchase low-sodium tomato juice, fruit in its own juice, and tuna packed in water.
- Use unsweetened applesauce and fruit purée as toppings for pancakes and waffles.
- Purchase eggs from range-fed chickens when possible.
- Flavor meats, grains, and vegetables with onion, garlic, and fresh herbs, which are excellent sources of phytochemicals.
- Roast your vegetables, which brings out their flavor and sweetness.
- When preparing wild game, reduce cooking time by up to 20 percent, since lean meat cooks faster than fattier cuts and can quickly become tough.
- Purchase unsalted nuts and seeds.
- When eating out, split an entrée and order extra servings of steamed vegetables or frequent the salad bar and focus on the fresh vegetables and fruits.

VARIETY IS THE KEY

"Eat a variety of food." You've heard this basic nutrition rule since you were a kid. Yet this recommendation carries a greater nutritional punch than we ever imagined. Our species survived, thrived, and evolved for millions of years because we ate a variety of foods, feasting on hundreds of different plants and animals. Research today repeatedly shows that the more varied our diets, the healthier and leaner we are, and the longer we can expect to live.

Variety is only healthful if it means lots of different fresh fruits, vegetables, nuts, seeds, legumes, and other plants. "The human body requires a wide variety of diverse plant foods, but that need has been distorted to mean wheat in a variety of ways," says Dr. George Armelagos.

Variety is most important for fruits, vegetables, and whole grains. These are the nutrient-packed foods that supply different fibers and the 12,000 phytochemicals on which your body evolved. Drink only orange juice and you'll miss out on the lycopene in tomatoes, the insoluble fiber in bran, the sulforaphane in broccoli, and the hundreds of sulfur compounds in garlic. Nutrient and phytochemical contents also vary depending on the species, where the plant is grown, and the time of year. In short, a tomato is not a tomato is not a tomato. So eat a variety of them. Variety is less important for meat and milk as long as all choices are low in saturated fat. Fish is an excellent source of the omega-3 fats not found in poultry breast, so a few servings of fish, especially fatty fish, should be included in your weekly diet.

How do you know if you're eating a varied diet? Is ten different foods each day enough or do you need twenty or thirty? One study from the American Dietetic Association attempted to answer this question by asking forty-eight people to record their food intakes. They found that those people who included at least seventy-one to eighty-three different foods in their diets during the two-week study had the highest vitamin C intakes, lowest sugar and salt intakes, and slightly lower saturated fat intakes compared to people who ate fewer than fifty-eight different foods. Keep a record of what you eat for any four days (include one weekend day) to check the level of variety in your diet. Use the box on pages 113–14, How Varied Is Your Diet?, to tally your results.

THOSE LITTLE CAVE HABITS

If lack of knowledge is the reason you overeat or choose the wrong things, then the answer is easy—start taking this nutrition thing seriously.

1. *Get fat-free savvy.* "What a fat-free cookie loses in fat, it gains in sugar; consequently, most fat-free desserts have about the same calories as regular ones," warns Dr. Adam Drewnowski. Fat-free cream cheese might be lower in calories, but not if you slather three times as much on a bagel. Use fat-free versions of anything sweet or creamy sparingly.

2. *Read labels.* Look for foods that supply no more than 3 grams of fat for every 100 calories. Also, note serving size, which might be unrealistically small, giving the false impression that the food is low in calories. Avoid products that contain hydrogenated vegetable oils and margarine (high in trans fatty acids), butter, or any vegetable oil other than olive or canola oils.

3. *Watch those portions.* We've become accustomed to gigantic servings. A 2-ounce bagel is now a 500-calorie, 4- to 7-ounce meal. The local deli heaps 6 ounces of turkey on your sandwich, not the 3 ounces considered a serving. "You are better off deciding what you want to eat, then putting an entire serving on a plate," says Dr. Barbara Rolls. "That way you get the full range of information on how much you're eating and are less likely to overdo it."

4. *Never socialize on an empty stomach.* People eat more when they're with friends and family. So have a healthful snack before a party, split an entrée when dining out, and don't mix alcohol with socializing, since even one drink breaks down the best of intentions, leaving you more likely to overeat.

5. *Do the grease-slick test.* Some foods don't come with labels, such as that bran muffin at the coffee shop or the doughnuts after church. But you usually can tell if something is high in fat by the slick feel in your mouth. If your doughnut leaves a grease stain on your fingers or a napkin, you can bet several teaspoons of fat (usually saturated or trans fatty acids) went into its making.

6. *Plan, plan, plan.* Bring foods with you. Stock the refrigerator with Stone Age items. Plan your meals in advance. "Unless you make a conscious decision to choose more fruits, vegetables, and whole grains, you will automatically and inevitably turn to high-fat, high-sugar items like cakes and cookies," cautions Dr. Drewnowski.

Fruits and Vegetables Rule

Origin Recommendation: eight to ten servings a day.

What's a serving? One piece of fruit or vegetable, 1 cup of raw, ½ cup cooked, 8 ounces juice.

How many servings of fresh fruits and vegetables did you eat yesterday? If you're like many Americans, you should double, even triple, that intake to meet the levels consumed by your ancient ancestors.

Our Paleolithic grandparents ate pounds of fresh fruits and vegetables, which are the real wonder foods of the Origin Diet. With the exception of avocados, olives, and coconut, fruits and vegetables have no fat, cholesterol, or sodium. They are the most nutrient-packed foods in the diet. In addition, they are loaded with water and fiber, but few calories (a heaping bowlful of greens supplies only 30 calories!), so they fill us up without filling us out—the perfect foods for people concerned about their waistlines. Studies repeatedly show that people who consume diets loaded with fresh fruits and vegetables are also the healthiest, with significantly lower disease rates and less risk for weight gain. It's vegetables and fruit in the Origin Diet that fill you up, so you don't feel hungry or deprived even though you're eating fewer calories and much less fat.

The good news is that it's never too late to enjoy the health-enhancing benefits of these nutritious foods, since improvements in health risks are noted within weeks of adding more fruits and vegetables to the diet. In short, *boosting your intake of fruits and vegetables to at least eight, and preferably ten servings a day is the best thing you can do for your health and your waistline.*

Sneaking those extra servings of vegetables and fruit into your daily diet is easy! Check out the box on pages 135–36 for some ideas. Also, consume more vegetables than fruit, since excessive fruit intake could cause digestive tract upsets and can temporarily aggravate blood triglycerides in people prone to elevated blood fats and heart disease.

EAT YOUR VEGETABLES!

Including eight to ten servings of fruits and vegetables in your daily diet isn't as difficult as it might first appear. Start slow, adding one extra serving a day. Then gradually increase this intake over several months.

- Include two servings of fruits and/or vegetables at every meal and snack. People on the Origin Diet have lost up to thirty pounds following this one guideline alone!
- Purée fresh fruit, such as apricots, blueberries, or peaches, and use as a topping on pancakes and waffles.
- Add vegetables to omelets.
- Feast on meal salads, by piling spinach or romaine lettuce on a plate and topping with grilled chicken breast or Cajun salmon.
- Mix chopped celery, grapes, apple, or dried cranberries into chicken salad.
- Make ice cubes of fruit purée to drop into cold drinks.
- Make fruit salsa with mango, peaches, pineapple, or papaya.
- Chop or grate zucchini or carrots into spaghetti sauce, chili, lasagna, or stews.
- Add puréed cooked vegetables, such as cauliflower, broccoli, or carrots, to soups and stews.

- Drink tomato juice, carrot juice, or V8 juice instead of soda pop.
- Try one new vegetable every week.
- Microwave a sweet potato for a snack.
- Add dried fruit to stuffings and rice dishes.
- Serve melon, grapefruit, fruit salad, gazpacho, or vegetable dishes as appetizers.
- Poach pears, bake apples, or freeze berries for desserts.
- Add edible flowers, such as geraniums, nasturtiums, violets, orange blossoms, and squash blossoms to salads.
- Try vegetables in different forms: raw, steamed, grilled, baked, sautéed in chicken broth, etc.
- Double your normal portion of any vegetable (except French fries or iceberg lettuce!).
- Add chopped tomatoes, fresh cilantro, and red onions to burritos and tacos.
- Add leftover vegetables to soups.
- Stock the freezer with plain, frozen vegetables for quick-fix meals.
- At salad bars, load the plate with dark green lettuce, raw vegetables, beans, and a little fresh fruit. Skip anything with mayonnaise, whipped cream, or oil.

IS FRESH BEST?

Fresh, frozen, or canned—which is more nutritious? While fresh-picked produce straight from your garden is best, it's more important that you eat more vegetables than it is whether they are fresh, frozen, or canned. Besides, fresh is only better if it's really fresh. Fresh produce that sits on the produce shelf for days or in your refrigerator all week often is less nutritious than frozen or canned vegetables, which are processed within hours of harvesting. For example, up to 58 percent of the vitamin C is lost in fresh green beans within three days of picking, while frozen green beans lose only about 20 percent of their vitamin C during processing.

Your best bet for maximizing the vitamin content of your vegetables is to

- Buy fresh and use them quickly. (Ancient foragers usually consumed gathered foods within hours of gathering and with minimal processing!)
- Keep your refrigerator at 40°F or below.
- If you can't guarantee that fresh produce is really fresh, then choose plain frozen vegetables or canned (without salt).
- Minimize chopping, since nutrients are lost in proportion to the surface area that is exposed.
- Cook vegetables in a small amount of liquid and only until crisp-tender.
- Use leftover liquids from the can or from cooking. Add to soups or stews.
- Include both raw and cooked vegetables in your daily diet.

WAXES, SPRAYS, AND PESTICIDES: ARE YOU GETTING TOO MUCH?

Pesticides are now part of our environment. There's no getting away from them, but we can reduce our exposure. Following the twelve Original Dozen will lower your pesticide exposure. Studies show that healthful diets based on whole grains, lots of fresh fruits and vegetables, legumes, and low-fat milk products consumed for at least three years lower the concentration of many pesticides in the body. Researchers at Tufts University School of Medicine in Boston report that consuming soy products inhibits pesticide-induced tumor growth by up to 50 percent. To limit your exposure to pesticides:

- Buy United States–grown organic produce, milk, and other products. Produce coming into the United States from other countries can contain illegal residues or levels of pesticides not allowed in this country. These foods are the ones to limit or avoid, if possible.
- Remove wax coatings. Waxes used to seal in moisture and keep produce fresh also seal in pesticides. Even organic produce uses waxes, such as beeswax and carnauba wax. To remove, wash fruits and vegetables with a mild soap solution. Rinse well.
- Peel conventional produce.

- Eat a low-fat diet of minimally processed foods. Keep in mind that pesticide residues also are found in meat, poultry, fish, butter, grains, and other foods. You can cut down on your risk by removing the fat, since that's where many pesticides are concentrated.
- Include soy products in your daily menu.

Regardless of the pesticide controversy, fresh fruits and vegetables are the most nutritious foods in the diet and should be consumed in greater quantities whether or not they're organic, homegrown, or grown by conventional methods.

ORGANIC VERSUS CONVENTIONAL—
WHICH IS BETTER?

Should you buy organic produce? The answer to that question depends on your reasons behind the purchase. If you are concerned about the environment, then yes, buy organic, since organic farming is much gentler on the land. Organic farming is much less harmful to the environment than conventional farming, reducing both the pesticide residues in food and the land, as well as reducing the contamination of our water supplies. Conventional farming pollutes water with pesticide runoff, degrades topsoil, and uses nonrenewable energy resources. In contrast, organic farming releases few chemicals into the environment, enhances soil quality, and encourages biodiversity of crops, thus protecting our natural resources. So, while organic produce is more costly on an immediate and personal level, it might be cost-effective for future generations.

If you're buying organic because you think it's more nutritious, then the answer is not so clear. Organic soil is healthier, so the produce grown in it should be more nutritious. Unfortunately, there is little research to support this assumption. Vitamin contents are similar, since plants make these nutrients, but minerals are absorbed from the ground, so plants can vary in their content of some of these nutrients, such as iodine, chromium, and selenium. Even when organic produce is found to contain more nutrients than conventionally grown produce, the differences are small and insignificant compared to variations in the weather and natural mineral contents of different soils. You get a much bigger nutritional bang for your buck in buying vine-ripened, very fresh produce, using fresh produce quickly, or growing your own than you do simply buying organic produce.

Fare Game/Wild Choices

Origin recommendation: one to two 3-ounce servings daily, supplemented with other protein-rich foods, such as legumes, nuts, seeds, and soy.

What's a serving? 3 ounces, or about the size of a deck of cards or the palm of your hand; 1 ounce nuts (approximately 3 tablespoons); 2 tablespoons nut butters; 4 ounces tofu; ¾ cup cooked dried beans and peas.

Up until the twentieth century, wild game was still available from the local butcher. Today, the meats that most resemble wild game and that are easily available have dwindled to poultry breast meat, shellfish, and fish. The latter two choices also supply the omega-3 fatty acids, so they should be included often in the weekly diet. Eggs are natural to our evolution; however, people with heart disease or diabetes should limit whole eggs or use egg substitutes or egg whites instead. Extra-lean red meat that contains 7 percent or less fat by weight can be included on occasion, such as once a week. Meats alien to our bodies include red meat from domesticated animals (beef, pork, lamb), dark poultry meat, bacon, sausage, and luncheon meats and hot dogs.

Some wild game, such as quail, pheasant, buffalo, elk, wild boar, ostrich, and antelope, is showing up on restaurant menus and in gourmet catalogs. Organic meat products from animals raised without antibiotic-laced feed or growth hormones and fed on lands free of chemical pesticides and fertilizers are also now commercially available. Even this game is farm raised, so its nutritional content is not an exact replacement of the meat on which we evolved, but is a close replica when affordable.

Extra-lean meats require tender loving care in preparation to avoid overcooking, which toughens the meat. Marinate these meats to tenderize and add flavor. Chicken breast, for example, is quite tender if seared on a hot grill to seal in moisture and then finished on low heat. Evolutionary styles of cooking include stewing, roasting, braising, baking, grilling, steaming, and boiling.

Grilling meat can produce cancer-causing substances called polycyclic aromatic hydrocarbons, which are formed in the smoke that coats grilled food when fat from the meat drops onto the hot coals. Other cancer-causing substances, heterocyclic amines (HCAs), form when muscle meat is cooked too quickly at high temperatures. You can reduce the formation of these harmful compounds by marinating meat before grilling, which reduces HCAs by 99 percent. Also, precook meat in a microwave for five to fifteen minutes (depending on the amount and type of meat) before grilling. Wrap meat in foil to reduce smoke exposure when possible, or cover the grill with foil and poke holes in it to let fat drip away (coat with vegetable spray to keep fish from sticking). Also, grill over medium, not hot, heat and avoid charring or blackening.

Other than fatty fish, such as salmon or mackerel, it is difficult to consume the level of omega-3s found in our ancient ancestors' diets. Fortunately, commercial products fortified with these fats are now available. For example, some eggs and bottled spaghetti sauce are enriched with omega-3s. A tablespoon of caviar contains 1 gram of omega-3s for only 40 calories! Flaxseed meal and oil contain a type of omega-3 called alpha linolenic acid; however, these omega-3s are not as effective as the ones found in fish oil in lowering blood triglyceride levels and heart disease risk.

Other protein-rich sources in our evolutionary diets included legumes and nuts. These options are high in vitamins, minerals, protein, and fiber, as well as a wealth of phytochemicals, such as isoflavones, ellagic acid, phenolic compounds, and flavonoids. Add nuts to salads, rice dishes, and fruit dishes. Several times a week include bean dishes, such as split pea soup, chili, fat-free refried bean burritos, or black beans and rice. Add beans to chili, make fat-free bean dip, serve beans as a side dish, or order bean-based soups at restaurants.

BROWN BAG LUNCHES

You can bring your lunch to work even if your office doesn't have a refrigerator. Just make it the night before and refrigerate to allow time for thorough chilling. You can even freeze sandwiches, but be sure to pack fat-free mayonnaise, lettuce, and tomatoes separately, since they don't freeze well. Use a small insulated bag or cooler, and put in a freeze-pack insert or cold drink to help keep everything cool.

Brown Bag Sandwiches, Burritos, and Wraps

Serve any of the following with fresh fruit such as grapes or orange slices, applesauce, a tossed salad, crunchy vegetables such as baby carrots with dip, dried nuts and fruits, a box of raisins, tomato or V8 juice, nonfat milk, soymilk, or yogurt, and/or a thermos of soup.

1. Turkey sandwich on whole wheat with mustard, 1 tablespoon fat-free cream cheese, 1 teaspoon sunflower seeds, and lettuce.
2. Tuna sandwich made with nonfat or low-fat mayonnaise and horseradish or celery seed (optional) on whole wheat with tomato and lettuce.
3. Salmon sandwich made with canned salmon, nonfat or low-fat mayonnaise, mustard, and lettuce on whole wheat.
4. Soy cheese sandwich made with fat-free soy cheese, mustard, lettuce, red onion slices, and tomato on whole wheat.
5. Peanut butter (or almond, cashew, or soy butter) with banana, sliced apple, apricots, or grated carrot on whole wheat.
6. Chicken salad sandwich made with chopped chicken breast mixed with nonfat mayonnaise, chopped celery, salt, and pepper with lettuce on whole wheat. (Curry is a nice spice for this sandwich.)
7. Hummus sandwich made with ½ cup hummus stuffed into a

---

whole wheat pita with chopped tomato, mint leaves, red onion slices, and/or cucumber slices.

8. Chicken breast with chutney made with 3 ounces sliced roasted chicken breast (remove the skin), 1 tablespoon Major Grey's chutney, and lettuce on whole wheat.

9. Cucumber and sprouts with fat-free cream cheese and 4 green olives on whole wheat bread.

10. Ricotta and nut sandwich: Mix ½ cup fat-free ricotta cheese, ¼ cup peanut butter, 2 teaspoons vanilla, ½ teaspoon cinnamon, and 1 tablespoon raisins. Place ½ Granny Smith apple, sliced, and ricotta-peanut butter mixture between two slices of whole wheat bread.

11. Creamy tortilla wrap: Spread the following into a whole wheat tortilla: fat-free cream cheese, bottled roasted red peppers, sliced red onion, and fresh basil leaves. Roll up.

12. Fill a pita: Stuff a whole wheat pita with sliced red onion, chopped red pepper, grated carrot, and black beans.

13. Yolkless egg salad: Mix 3 cooked egg whites with fat-free mayonnaise, 3 tablespoons chopped celery, 1 teaspoon fresh dill, and salt and pepper. Stuff into a whole wheat pita.

14. Garden or veggie burger with mustard, lettuce, and tomato on a whole wheat bun.

15. Spread Dijon mustard, 2 romaine lettuce leaves (cores removed), bottled roasted red peppers, and ¼ cup of store-bought tabbouleh on a whole wheat tortilla. Roll up firmly, slice diagonally into two pieces, and wrap in plastic wrap.

In a thermos

1. ½ of a 15-ounce can of low-fat turkey chili.

2. 1 can low-fat minestrone or vegetable soup, split pea soup, lentil soup, vegetarian chili.

3. Piña colada shake: Whip in a blender and pour into a thermos 1 frozen banana, ½ cup pineapple, 1 cup nonfat plain yogurt, ¼ teaspoon coconut extract, and ¼ cup nonfat milk.

4. Pack leftovers, such as spaghetti, stew, or a rice and chicken casserole.

Other Ideas

1. If you have a microwave at work, pack a low-fat frozen entrée, such as Weight Watchers Smart Ones Chicken Français or Chicken Mirabella.
2. Cold plate: 2 ounces sliced turkey breast, 2 slices fat-free soy cheese, 6 whole wheat crackers or 2 slices whole wheat bread, and 1 cup sliced raw vegetables with 2 tablespoons low-fat dip or dressing.
3. Skewer fresh fruit pieces for a fruit kabob.
4. Pack baked tortilla chips with fat-free refried bean dip and salsa.
5. Mini pizza: Use easy-to-pack ingredients to make a pizza at work: whole wheat English muffin or a whole wheat pita, pizza sauce, grated soy cheese, and veggies.
6. Grab a sweet potato as you bolt out the door in the morning. Microwave at work for 5 to 10 minutes and sprinkle with cinnamon (keep on hand in your desk). Grab a carton of low-fat or nonfat milk and a piece of fruit from the vending machine.
7. Open a can of chickpeas, rinse, toss with 1 teaspoon olive oil, 1 teaspoon red wine or balsamic vinegar, and a dash of salt and paprika. Place in container for a quick-fix lunch served with fresh fruit, whole wheat crackers, milk, and/or yogurt.
8. Meat salads: Mix chopped chicken breast, sliced red grapes, chopped apple, chopped celery, raisins, and diced red onion with nonfat mayonnaise, a dash of lemon, and salt and pepper. Pack chopped romaine lettuce in one container and the chicken mixture in another. Combine at lunch.
9. Meal salads: Toss 1 cup whole wheat couscous with 1 teaspoon curry powder, $\frac{1}{4}$ cup each slivered almonds, raisins, and chopped dried apricots. Mix with 1 tablespoon olive oil and $\frac{1}{4}$ teaspoon lemon juice. Serve with the chickpeas from idea #7 above.
10. Taco salad: $\frac{2}{3}$ cup canned pinto or kidney beans, 1 ounce grated

fat-free soy cheese, 1 diced tomato, ¼ cup grated carrots,
3 tablespoons diced green pepper, 2 cups chopped leaf lettuce,
1 corn tortilla toasted and broken into chips, and salsa on the side.

Sweets

1. Stick an almond into a dried date or prune. Pack four of these in your lunch.
2. Blend equal parts fat-free cottage cheese and nonfat milk. Sweeten with honey, nutmeg, cinnamon, and/or vanilla and serve as a dip with fresh fruit.
3. Apple Crisp: Peel a medium apple halfway down from top. Remove core almost to the bottom, leaving a 1-inch opening at top. Microwave for 4 minutes, or until apple is tender. Mix 1 tablespoon Grape-Nuts cereal and 1 tablespoon all-fruit jam (raspberry, apricot, or strawberry are good) and pack mixture into apple opening. Microwave for 1 minute.
4. Fill celery stalks with peanut butter and top with dried cranberries.
5. Make low-fat muffins with honey and pack one in your lunch.
6. Fill ½ cantaloupe with 1 cup nonfat plain yogurt flavored with 2 teaspoons honey and 1 teaspoon lemon zest. Wrap tightly in plastic wrap and place upright in insulated lunch box.
7. Citrus confetti: Mix 1 peeled and chopped grapefruit, 1 peeled and chopped orange, 1 peeled and chopped tangerine, 2 tablespoons chopped pecans, ⅓ cup orange juice, 2 tablespoons honey, and chopped fresh mint for a garnish. (Makes about 3 cups.)

How Much Water?

Origin recommendation: At least eight glasses of water a day.
What's a serving? 8 ounces.

From water came all life on this earth. We reflect those ultra-ancient origins by the fact that our bodies are up to 70 percent water. Water is the most important nutrient; we can survive for up to two months without food, but only seven to eight days without water. Water must have been abundant during our evolution, because our bodies never developed a system for conserving it. We lose about two to three quarts daily, even more if we exercise or work in hot climates. That means you, like all of your ancient ancestors, need to take in about a gallon of fluid every day to replace these losses.

Thirst is a poor indicator of fluid needs. To make sure you get enough, drink

1. twice as much water as it takes to quench your thirst,
2. at least eight glasses of water daily or one cup of water for every twenty pounds of body weight.

You can count fruit juices and bottled water in your tally, but not beverages unknown in ancient times, such as coffee, soda pop, or alcohol. Green tea, a natural beverage loaded with cancer-fighting phytochemicals, is another way to add fluids. To reach your quota, fill a pitcher with your daily allotment of water and keep it on your desk at work or the kitchen counter at home. Your goal is clearly marked and the empty container lets you know you've met that goal. Bring a filled water bottle with you in the car, take ten gulps of water every time you pass a water fountain, and drink two to three glasses of water during restaurant meals.

Water also is an ancient secret for weight loss and control of sweet cravings. Many people who have adopted the Origin Diet comment that as they increased their water intakes, their sweet cravings stopped. Patricia said, "Many times I think I want to eat something sweet, when in fact I'm really thirsty and the water satisfies me."

Are tea, coffee, and alcohol allowed in the Origin Diet? There is no evidence that moderate amounts of tea or coffee (i.e., up to three cups a day) are harmful to our evolutionary bodies. Even small amounts of alcohol are tolerated, probably because fruits naturally fermented in ancient times and so were available in modest amounts. Two to three alcoholic beverages a week (one drink = 6 ounces wine, 12 ounces beer,

1 ounce liquor) or a little alcohol used in cooking is within the Origin guidelines.

New Age Versus Stone Age

"Planning. That has been the most important habit I've learned. Eating well is a breeze when I plan ahead."—Sharon

The secret to returning to your dietary roots and sticking with this way of eating is twofold:

1. Plan ahead.
2. Keep healthful foods handy.

Stock the kitchen with quick-fix Origin basics, such as canned beans, canned tomatoes, nonstick cooking sprays, brown rice mixes, whole wheat tortillas, whole grains, fresh fruit, frozen plain vegetables, honey mustard, olive oil, cilantro, whole wheat bread, orange juice, skinless chicken breast, sweet potatoes, and other suggested foods on the Origin Shopping List, pages 158–60. Throw out the butter, bacon, potato chips, ice cream, and soda pop. You'll be tempted to eat these non-Origin foods if you keep them around, especially in the first few weeks.

Always, *I mean always,* bring food with you (you need to eat about every four hours). If you bolt from the house without a food stash, I guarantee you'll wind up eating what's available from a vending machine or a fast-food restaurant, and we all know they don't stock healthful items! (See below for some good alternatives.)

Looking for Healthful Alternatives?

TYPICAL FOODS	STONE AGE ALTERNATIVES
Cheese	Fat-free cheese, soy cheeses
Jam/jellies	All-fruit spread
White or "wheat" bread	100 percent whole wheat bread

TYPICAL FOODS	STONE AGE ALTERNATIVES
Beef, pork, lamb	Skinless poultry breast meat, all fish and shellfish, wild game, cooked dried beans and peas, tofu and soy products
Ground beef	Ground turkey breast
Milk	Calcium-fortified soymilk
French fries	Baked sweet potato fries
Hamburger	Turkey burger made with ground turkey breast, sliced tomato, lettuce, mustard
White rice	Brown rice, wild rice, quinoa, bulgur
Alcohol	Fruit juice, nonalcoholic fruit-based beverages
Eggs	Whole eggs (limit to five per week, preferably from range-fed hens), egg whites, egg substitute
Potato chips and other snack foods	Nuts, soy nuts
Commercial peanut butter (high in sugar)	Natural peanut butter, other nut butters, natural soy butter
Sugar, high-fructose corn syrup, brown sugar	Honey, dried fruit, fruit juice concentrate
Canned fruit in heavy syrup	Canned fruit in own juice
Frozen vegetables in sauce	Plain frozen vegetables
Chicken with skin	Chicken breast without skin
Canned spaghetti sauce (high in salt or fat)	Tomato paste, tomato sauce, canned tomatoes, bottled fat-free spaghetti sauce, fresh tomatoes
Egg noodles	Whole wheat noodles, spaghetti squash
Butter and margarine	Olive oil, canola oil, fat-free butter substitutes
Oil for sautéing	Chicken or vegetable broth
Mayonnaise on sandwiches	Fat-free mayonnaise, mustard, salsa, roasted red peppers, canned chilies, pickled ginger, or other spices
Syrup on your pancakes or waffles	Puréed fresh fruit sweetened with honey

I can't emphasize enough the importance of these two rules. You will be successful only if you keep Origin foods with you. Take Susan, for example, who calls herself a bag lady because she brings bags of fruit and carrots with her everywhere. "I leave the bag on my desk at work and when I come through to grab a new folder for the next meeting, I grab a couple of carrots or an orange slice and eat them on the way. If it wasn't for those bags, I'd either not eat at all and be ravenous at dinner or eat all the wrong foods."

WHAT ABOUT FAT?

Origin recommendation: When you include only natural fats in the diet, you can stop worrying about fat grams.

What's a serving? One ounce nuts, 1 tablespoon olive oil, ¼ avocado, 3 ounces salmon or other fatty fish.

It's the saturated fat that's alien to our bodies, increasing disease risk. Throw out the butter, cream, margarine, red meats, processed meats, and fatty bacon and luncheon meats. Toss the processed foods, which range from potato chips and cookies to fried fast foods and doughnuts, and which contain saturated fats or trans fatty acids from hydrogenated vegetable oils.

Natural fats—those found in our diets since the dawn of humans— are essential for optimal health. Olives and olive oil, avocados, nuts, and omega-3 fatty acid–rich fish are not only safe, they are needed by our bodies and our brains. Of course, that doesn't give us license to go overboard. These fats are just as calorie-concentrated as saturated fat and will add inches to our waistlines if consumed in excess. However, use a little common sense when it comes to serving size, then stop worrying about counting fat grams or eliminating natural fats and start enjoying the taste and textures of these healthful foods. If you follow the guidelines of the Origin Diet, you will automatically consume a diet that contains about 25 percent fat calories from the healthful fats, and is low in saturated fats.

Interestingly, your body will soon adapt to this new style of eating and the fatty foods that once sounded like treats, from cheese to chocolate, will lose their appeal. Sue summed it up when she said, "I find that my energy is more consistent now that I've been eating right. Previously, a stressful morning would find me looking for a fatty lunch. I still have stressful mornings, but a heavy lunch sounds like a punishment, not a reward."

THE CASE FOR WHOLE GRAINS

Origin recommendation: Focus on whole grains and starchy vegetables, such as sweet potatoes and corn. Include at least six servings of whole grains in your daily diet.

What's a serving? One slice of whole grain bread; ½ cup cooked whole grain cereal, brown rice, or whole grain pasta; 1 small whole grain tortilla; or ½ whole wheat English muffin, hamburger bun, 3-ounce bagel, ½ cup cooked starchy vegetable.

Our Paleolithic grandparents didn't eat a lot of grain and they certainly didn't grind grains into flour. But there is reason to include these nutritional gold mines in the Origin Diet. For one thing, grass seeds, like wheat or barley, were a part of our original diets. These wholesome plants are as natural as a sprig of parsley or a leaf of lettuce. It's only when we refine them, process them, and extract their fiber and nutrients that we turn them into nutritional wastelands, reducing their vitamin, mineral, fiber, and phytochemical contents to mere shadows of their former selves. "People did not evolve eating refined grains," says Dr. Walter Willett. "Highly processed grains appear to aggravate the glycemic load and increase the risk for diabetes; people are better off eating breads and cereals in their whole grain forms." You're also hard-pressed to reach the level of carbohydrate calories found in our ancestors' diets (about 45 percent to 50 percent of total calories) without including both root vegetables and whole grains.

Finally, numerous studies spanning decades of research show that whole grains and their fibers, phytochemicals (such as ferulic and caffeic acids and lignans), and vast vitamin and mineral contents help lower disease risk, boost our health, and possibly even trim our waistlines. Researchers at Harvard Medical School in Boston, who studied the effects of diet on health status in 75,521 women in the Nurses' Health Study, showed that women who consumed the most whole grains every day lowered their risk for heart disease by 33 percent. Whole grains also are associated with lowered cancer and diabetes risk.

Focus only on whole grains, not on refined fiber products. A lower disease risk is linked more to fiber-rich foods commonly found in ancient diets than to fiber itself. The mixture of both insoluble and soluble fibers from a variety of minimally processed foods is what our bodies evolved on and is what improves our health, which is a far cry from the bowl of processed bran added to an otherwise low-fiber diet.

Relying on commercially prepared "fiber" foods has other drawbacks. Many of the commercial foods advertised as high fiber actually have little to back up those claims. Bread labels that read "bran," "wheat berry," "multigrain," "seven-grain," "crunchy," "sprouted wheat," "organic," "stoneground," or "cracked wheat" usually contain more white flour than any of those ingredients. Often their wheaty appearance comes from caramel coloring, not natural grains. Or they combine white flour with wheat bran to give the appearance of a whole-grain product.

Other processed fiber products, from fiber bars and powders to bakery goods and crackers, also run the gamut from nutritious to junk food. "Wheat" usually means white flour, even if wheat shafts and baskets of grain decorate the package. Many of these commercial products also are high in fat, salt, or sugar. You must become a fiber sleuth and read labels for high-fiber, low-fat options. Here's what to look for:

- Select only wheat products, such as breads, ready-to-eat cereals, and tortillas, that are 100 percent whole wheat or that list whole-grain flours as the first ingredient on the label.

• Eat a variety of grains, including amaranth, barley, black japonica rice, brown rice, bulgur, cornmeal, millet, oats, quinoa, rye, soy flour, spelt, teff, triticale, wehani rice, wheat berries, and wild rice.

• Exceptions to the whole grain rule are toasted wheat germ, flaxseed meal, and oat bran, which are nutritional powerhouses. Add them to batters for muffins, pancakes, waffles, breads, and cookies. Mix into turkey breast meatloaves, sprinkle on top of cereal, and blend into smoothies. Also mix wheat germ with equal parts honey and nut butters for a sandwich spread.

• If you're not used to cooking with whole-grain flours, start with whole wheat pastry flour, which is ground to a finer texture and lighter consistency than unbleached white flour or whole wheat flours. Or, mix half unbleached white flour with half whole wheat.

• The more unprocessed the grain, the greater its fiber content. Whole wheat berries are higher in fiber than stone-ground whole wheat flour, which is higher in fiber than whole wheat pastry flour.

HUNTER-GATHERER SNACKS

For each snack, pick one to three items from column 1 and one item from column 2.

Column 1	*Column 2*
Fruit: Apple, applesauce (unsweetened), apricot, banana, berries, cherries, grapefruit, grapes, kiwi, mango, melons, nectarine, orange, papaya, peach, pear, pineapple, plum, quince, star fruit, tangerine, watermelon Serving: 1 piece of fruit or 1 cup	Nuts: Almonds, cashews, peanuts, pistachios Serving: 1 ounce or about 20 nuts Milk/Soy: Nonfat milk, yogurt, cheese. Calcium-fortified soy cheese or soymilk Serving: 1 cup, 1 ounce cheese

Column 1

Vegetable: Artichoke, asparagus, bean sprouts, broccoli, Brussels sprouts, cabbage, carrots, cauliflower, celery, cucumber, green beans, jicama, lettuce greens (salad), mushrooms, parsnips, pea pods, green peas, peppers, potato, pumpkin, spinach (salad), summer squash, sweet potato (baked), tomato
Serving: 1 vegetable (i.e., carrot), 1 cup raw or ½ cup cooked

Grains: Whole wheat bread, pita bread, English muffin, tortilla (fat-free), bagel, crackers, pretzel, or couscous salad, brown rice pudding, rice cakes, corn tortillas
Serving: 1 slice, ½ cup, 2 rice cakes, ½ English muffin, hamburger bun, bagel

Column 2

Meat/Beans: Extra-lean slice of turkey, chicken breast meat, split pea soup, lentil soup, chili beans, beans on a salad or on top of a corn tortilla, canned salmon or tuna (canned in water), hummus, eggs
Serving: 3 ounces meat or fish, ¾ cup beans, ½ cup hummus

Extras: Olives, avocado slices, honey
Serving: 5 olives, 2 avocado slices, 1 tablespoon honey

Suggestions

1. Soy cheese and crackers with a piece of fruit.
2. Hummus with whole wheat pita bread and baby carrots.
3. One cup nonfat milk warmed and sprinkled with nutmeg. Serve with 1 soft whole wheat pretzel topped with Dijon mustard.
4. One cup nonfat plain yogurt sweetened with honey and served with a piece of fruit.
5. Deviled egg made with fat-free mayonnaise, mustard, salt, pepper, and paprika to taste. Serve with baby carrots, a piece of fruit, and/or whole wheat crackers.

6. Drain a can of chickpeas, toss with 1 teaspoon olive oil and bake until crisp, shaking the cookie sheet several times during baking to prevent sticking (about 1 hour at 350°F). Serve with crackers and fruit.

7. Top artichoke bottoms (from a can) with a mixture of shrimp or crabmeat, nonfat mayonnaise, a pinch of red pepper, tarragon, and salt. Serve with crunchy vegetables.

8. Mix chutney and fat-free cream cheese, then use as a topping for whole wheat crackers. Serve with fresh fruit.

9. Potatoes à la Hummus: Boil baby red potatoes. Cool. Scoop out a teaspoon-sized hollow and fill with hummus (store-bought or homemade). Sprinkle with paprika or chopped mint.

10. A low-fat bran muffin with apple butter. Serve with a glass of nonfat milk and a piece of fruit.

11. Mix shredded carrots with raisins and nonfat salad dressing and pile on top of a slice of toasted whole wheat bread.

12. Top 1 slice whole wheat toast with 2 tablespoons fat-free ricotta cheese and a dash of cinnamon and nutmeg. Broil until bubbly. Serve with a piece of fruit.

13. Peaches and Cream: Combine 2 tablespoons fat-free cream cheese with 1 teaspoon honey and 1 fresh peach, peeled and chopped. Spread on whole wheat bread.

14. Tortilla wrap: Fill one whole wheat tortilla with 2 tablespoons fat-free refried beans, ¼ cup chopped spinach leaves, 1 slice mozzarella-style soy cheese, and 2 tablespoons salsa. Roll tightly.

15. Sticks 'n' Stones Salad: Place one cup steamed green beans and ½ cup cherry tomatoes in a bowl and toss with ½ teaspoon olive oil, 1 tablespoon champagne vinegar, ½ teaspoon Dijon mustard, 2 tablespoons chopped parsley, and a dash of salt. Serve with a glass of milk.

16. Trail mix made with 2 tablespoons dried cranberries, 2 table-spoons sunflower seeds, and ¼ cup whole wheat cereal. Serve with nonfat yogurt or milk.

17. Large baked potato topped with ½ cup steamed spinach, diced tomatoes, and fresh herbs.
18. Chewy 'n' Sweet: Wrap dried apricots around five to ten almonds. Serve with nonfat milk.

THE CASE FOR MILK

Origin recommendation: Two to three servings daily of nonfat milk products or calcium-fortified soymilk.

What's a serving? Eight-ounce glass of nonfat milk or soymilk, 2 cups fat-free cottage cheese, 1 cup nonfat plain yogurt, or 1 ounce fat-free cheese.

Milk has graced dining tables for only about ten thousand years, so there is no evidence that adults must drink milk. However, we're hard-pressed to meet our calcium and vitamin D needs without it. For example, milk supplies up to 75 percent of many adults' calcium intake. Take away the milk and you must consume 35 cups of cooked collard greens, 100 cups of regular soymilk, or 16 ounces of canned salmon every day. The only viable alternative is calcium-fortified foods, such as soymilk or orange juice. Except for milk and fortified soymilk, no other foods are reliable sources of vitamin D (cheese, yogurt, and cottage cheese aren't fortified with this vitamin).

Most women fall short of the daily calcium recommendation of 1,000 to 1,200 milligrams, while our ancient ancestors averaged up to 1,900 milligrams daily. An overwhelming amount of research shows that the high calcium intakes of our ancestors protected them against age-related bone loss and fractures. Calcium is the key ingredient here, but since milk is the best dietary source of this mineral, it makes sense to include nonfat milk products in the daily diet.

For these reasons, the Stone Age diet has been modernized to fit our Modern Age lifestyles. Include at least two to three low-fat calcium-rich foods in your daily menu, including nonfat milk products and calcium-fortified products like soymilk or orange juice. Take a calcium supplement and a multiple supplement that contains vitamin D to fill in the gaps on the days when you don't eat perfectly. Other ways to boost calcium intake: Prepare oatmeal and rice in milk, spread nonfat ricotta cheese on toast for a snack, buy extra-firm tofu (it has more calcium than softer tofu), prepare creamed soups with nonfat milk, use nonfat yogurt for dips, use fat-free cream cheese and sour cream, add nonfat powdered milk to recipes such as soups and casseroles, and snack on fat-free string cheese.

MORE EVOLUTIONARY QUICK TRICKS

- Make the produce section your main grocery-shopping attraction. Load the cart with a wide variety of produce and try a new fruit or vegetable at least once a week.
- Sweeten nonfat plain yogurt with honey, nuts, dried fruits, fresh fruit, or lemon/orange peel.
- Read labels and steer clear of foods that provide more than 30 percent of calories from fat, have more saturated fat than unsaturated fat, or are made with hydrogenated vegetable oils.
- Add tofu to soups, wraps, stir fries, veggie burgers, and sandwiches. Try to drink calcium-fortified soymilk at least three times a week.
- Add nonfat yogurt to smoothies to boost intake of healthful bacteria so abundant in our ancient ancestors' diets.
- Add flaxseed meal or wheat germ to pancake batters, muffin mixes, and hot cereal to boost omega-3 fatty acids (in the case of flax) and iron, zinc, B vitamins, magnesium, and fiber (in the case of wheat germ).
- Always choose spinach and romaine lettuce over head lettuce to boost fiber, vitamins, minerals, and phytochemical intakes.

- Experiment with cooked dried beans and peas. Add kidney beans to soups and burritos, make dips and vegetable spreads from cooked yellow split peas, and use spiced lentils as a side dish. A half cup of beans supplies 8 grams of fiber, 22 grams of protein, and hefty doses of iron, zinc, B vitamins, and saponins, phytochemicals that lower your risk for heart disease and cancer.
- Use herbs and spices to entice your tastebuds. The added benefit is that herbs, such as basil, marjoram, thyme, and rosemary, and ginger and garlic contain phytochemicals that lower cancer and heart-disease risk.
- Sprinkle sunflower seeds on a sandwich or in a wrap to give it crunch, slivered almonds on vegetables, or olives on anything.
- Try juicing your fruits and vegetables. Start out with the basic—carrots, celery, and apple—then venture into more exotic combinations, such as carrot, ginger, parsley, and garlic. The combinations are endless!
- Cut sweet potatoes into ½-inch strips and roast for a tasty alternative to French fries.

SATISFYING YOUR SWEET TOOTH

Origin recommendation: Sweeten foods with honey, maple syrup, date sugar.

What's a serving? Limit daily intake to 6 teaspoons.

Our bodies haven't evolved a system to handle the 20 teaspoons or more of sugar that we consume in sweets, baked goods, processed foods, and soda pop. These foods also replace the foods, nutrients, and phytochemicals on which our bodies thrive. For these reasons, you won't find sugar in the Origin Diet. You will find honey, maple syrup, date sugar, and fruit purées. The only precaution is to avoid giving honey to children under two years old, since even tiny amounts of a bacteria occasionally found in honey can cause a dangerous infection called botulism in very small children.

Wean yourself from sweets by slowly cutting back on sugar in recipes:

Use honey instead of sugar in favorite foods and use fresh fruits and fruit purées. Honey can turn a nutritious snack into a dessert. For example:

- Sprinkle chopped pecans over plain nonfat yogurt and drizzle with honey.
- Spread nonfat ricotta cheese on a whole wheat bagel, sprinkle with walnuts, and top with a drizzle of honey.
- Mix honey and nonfat sour cream and use as a topping on fresh fruits or berries.

People who have adopted the Origin Diet say their sweet tooth subsides within weeks. They don't want or crave added sugars and find natural foods more flavorful and satisfying. "I noticed a big difference in my cravings for sweets within about two weeks of starting the diet," said Emma. "Thank goodness! Now I yearn for a piece of fruit; regular desserts are just too sweet." By the second week of being on the diet, Susan was amazed to find she rarely needed her daily soda pop. "I can't believe that I only had one cola this week, and I didn't even really think about it. My other cravings, like for cheese, are pretty much gone, too!"

Fast-Food Cooking

Does trying to fit healthy eating into an already overbooked schedule seem like a no-win situation? Who has time to cut up vegetables, boil beans, or make a salad when it's so much easier to order take-out pizza?

One of the most common nutrition myths is that eating healthfully takes more time. But time is no longer an issue when it comes to eating well, especially with the wealth of new, healthful convenience foods. "You don't need to eat a hot meal or even cook to be healthy," says Evelyn Tribole, M.S., R.D., author of *Stealth Health* (Viking Press, 1999). In fact, with a well-stocked kitchen (see box on pages 158–60), it takes less time to prepare a low-fat, nutritious Origin meal than it does for that take-out order to arrive. It does take a change in mind-set and a little planning up front.

THE ORIGIN SHOPPING LIST

This is not a complete list, but gives ideas for shopping the Origin way. Use this sheet as a master copy. Keep a copy posted in the kitchen to circle needed items, then take the completed list with you when you shop. Shopping tips: Shop from a list, don't shop when hungry, and read labels!

The Produce Section

All fruits, including apple, apricots, bananas, berries, cantaloupe, casaba melon, cherries, grapefruit, grapes, kiwi, kumquats, honeydew melon, nectarines, oranges, papayas, peaches, pears, pineapple, plums, pomegranate, quince, starfruit, tangerine, watermelon
Other: _____

All vegetables, including artichoke, asparagus, bean sprouts, beets, broccoli, Brussels sprouts, cabbage, carrots, cauliflower, celery, cilantro, cucumber, chard, collards, corn, dandelion greens, eggplant, garlic, ginger, green beans, herbs, jicama, kale, leeks, lettuce, mushrooms, mustard greens, okra, onions, parsley, parsnips, pea pods, peas, green peppers, potato, pumpkin, rhubarb, rutabaga, spinach, summer squash, sweet potato, tomato, turnip greens, winter squash, yam
Other: _____

Breads and Crackers, Whole Grain Only
(check labels and avoid products with hydrogenated vegetable oils)

Bread, bagels, English muffins, pitas, tortillas: oatmeal, pumpernickel, rye, and whole wheat, 100 percent whole wheat crackers, corn tortillas, rice cakes made from brown rice
Other: _____

The Dairy Case

Nonfat milk, nonfat plain yogurt, buttermilk (made from nonfat milk), fat-free cheeses, soy cheeses, fat-free sour cream, fat-free cream cheese, eggs, egg substitute
Other: _____

The Meat Department

White meat, chicken and turkey; ground turkey breast
All seafood
Other: _____

Dry Goods

Buttermilk (dry), powdered nonfat milk, flour (whole wheat, rye, soy), dried beans and peas, whole grain pasta, brown rice, quick-cooking brown rice, cornmeal, quinoa, bulgur, barley, wheat berries, wild rice, millet, whole wheat couscous, nuts, unsalted and raw or dry-roasted
Other: _____

Canned Goods

Applesauce (no sugar added), fruit (canned in own juice), artichoke hearts (water-packed), beans (kidney, black, garbanzo), carrot juice, evaporated nonfat milk, fruit cocktail (canned in own juice), 100 percent fruit juices (avoid white grape juice and pear juice), mandarin oranges (juice packed), peaches (canned in own juice), peanut butter, pear (canned in own juice), pineapple chunks (canned in own juice), salmon (canned), soups, low-fat soymilk (preferably fortified with calcium, vitamin D, and vitamin B_{12}), spaghetti sauce (fat free), tomato juice, tomato paste, tomato sauce, tuna (water-packed), plain vegetables
Other: _____

Breakfast Cereals *(Check labels for brands with less than 2 grams fat and little or no sugar in ingredients list)*

Cooked: Oatmeal, barley, seven-grain
Ready-to-eat, low-fat, whole grain: Grape-Nuts, Shredded Wheat, Nutri-Grain, granola (only if fat-free or oil listed on label is canola oil, and if low in added sugars)
Wheat germ
Other: _____

Frozen Foods

Frozen fruit ice, frozen orange juice concentrate, frozen fruit (strawberries, blueberries)
Plain frozen vegetables
Waffles, whole wheat
Other: _____

Snack Items

Dried fruit, nuts and seeds, popcorn (plain), potato chips (oven-baked, fat-free), whole wheat pretzels, tortilla chips (oven-baked, fat-free), soy nuts
Other: _____

Herbs, Oils, and Condiments

Active dry yeast, all-fruit jam, baking powder, baking soda, cornstarch, herbs and spices, lemon juice, mustard, speciality mustards, no-fat salad dressings, oil (olive or canola), salsa, unflavored gelatin, vanilla, vinegar, honey, chili oil, tahini (sesame seed paste), speciality vinegars, capers, horseradish, clam juice, Tabasco, lime juice, chili sauce
Other: _____

How can you eat well without living in the kitchen? It's simple—just follow any or all of the following quick-fix tips:

- *Keep nutritious foods readily available.* Clean and store enough raw vegetables to supply meals and snacks for up to three days. (Or purchase vegetables, salad greens, or fresh fruit already washed and cut.) Freeze an extra loaf of whole wheat bread, stock extra cans of kidney beans, fill the cookie jar with homemade trail mix made with nuts, dried fruits, and roasted soybeans.
- *Make more than you need.* When preparing a meal, cook extra chicken or brown rice, chop extra celery or green onions, grate extra carrots, or squeeze extra lemon juice and store in the refrigerator to use later in the week.
- *Prepare meals in quantity.* Make a big pot of soup or a stew, spaghetti, lasagna, casseroles, chicken or bean wraps, or sauces that are great for lunches or dinners throughout the week, or to freeze in individual containers for later use.
- *Keep it simple.* "Unless you are a gourmet cook who loves to spend hours in the kitchen, avoid complicated recipes that require time, a lengthy list of ingredients, and fancy equipment," says Tribole.
- *Take advantage of nutritious quick-fix foods.* Purchase precut vegetables and fruits, bottled minced garlic or ginger, bottled lemon juice, frozen whole wheat waffles, preshredded cabbage, bagged lettuce or spinach, bulk bags of frozen skinned and boned chicken breasts, canned kidney beans, fat-free half and half, and boxed or premade hummus.
- *Use the microwave.* You can microwave a sweet potato in five minutes, heat up leftovers in seconds, and even precook chicken before placing it on the barbecue.

If you think that eating well requires a total revamp of your dietary habits, think again. More often, all it takes are a few minor changes in what, when, or how you eat, such as including two fruits and/or vegetables at every meal or snack, taking time to eat breakfast (which boosts energy and curbs uncontrollable hunger cravings later in the day), or paying attention to portion size. As one person said, "This way of eating is much easier than I thought it might be. I'm having fun exploring recipes and getting back to basics." If you're concerned that you don't have the time or energy, keep in mind that everyone who adopts this evolutionary eating plan reports a boost in energy. So, you'll have more motivation to go the extra mile and feel even better!

HOW TO CONVERT RECIPES AND MENUS

As you experiment with the Origin Diet, you're likely to find that most recipes are easily adapted to this new style of eating. Some recipes might require only modest changes, such as using nonfat milk instead of whole milk or substituting prune purée for the fat in an oatmeal cookie recipe. Other recipes might take some imagination, requiring several ingredient changes and some trial and error before you create a good alternative. The recipes most likely to fail the test are the ones heavily dependent on highly refined ingredients and sugar. The good news is that you will lose your taste for these foods within the first few weeks of adopting the Origin Diet.

Be adventuresome, like Katherine, who found that she was more satisfied on less food when that food had more flavor. "Foods taste better on this eating plan and they have a wider variety of flavors than my old diet. I find that I eat more often, but I'm satisfied with fewer calories."

As you cut back on the monotonous tastes of sweet or salt in highly processed foods, your tastebuds are reawakened to a world of other flavors, such as the earthy flavor of chickweed, the chicory-like taste of dandelion, the spinachy flavor of amaranth, or the dill-like taste of yarrow. Add new vegetables to your menu, such as bok choy, chayote, jicama, okra, taro root, or yucca root. Experiment with new seasonings, such as fresh ginger, saffron, horseradish, chipotle peppers in adobo sauce, red curry paste, red chili paste, fresh herbs, or orange zest (orange peel), and reduce your risk for cancer while you're exciting your tastebuds. See the Appendix and the recipe sections for a five-day meal plan, recipes, and suggestions for mix-and-match breakfasts, lunches, and dinners.

EVOLUTION AND VEGETARIAN DIETS

All of our ancestors—dating back hundreds of thousands of years—ate meat. Meat has been a key dietary ingredient in our evolution, but it is not an absolute necessity. Our bodies need a variety of nutrients, but fortunately they don't know or care where those nutrients are obtained. You can get the nine essential amino acids needed to build protein from an elk steak or from mixing black beans and brown rice. You can get the iron your red blood cells need from venison stew or from prunes, spinach, lentils, or a variety of plants.

One thing we do know is that vegetarian diets are much healthier than the typical westernized diet. Several studies show that America's 15 million vegetarians have much lower rates of cancer and hypertension, and up to a 50 percent lower risk for heart disease compared to the general public. They also have an easier time managing their weight and they live longer. In all fairness to carnivores, the real issue might not be the steak per se, but both the harmful effects of its saturated fat plus the absence of protective effects of other foods in the vegetarian diet. People who eat lots of fruits, legumes, vegetables, and whole grains— with or without meat—are at much lower risk for certain cancers and heart disease.

No studies have followed vegetarian kids through adulthood, so we don't know for sure whether starting young has added advantages. Adult obesity and heart disease have their roots in childhood, so many caring parents have reduced the fat and even gone vegetarian to spare their children from these fates. But even if vegetarian fare lowers heart-disease risk, many vegetarian diets fall short when it comes to meeting the high nutrient demands of growing bodies. "It's easiest to get enough of all the nutrients and calories when people eat a wide variety of wholesome foods. The more foods you eliminate from the diet, the greater is the likelihood of nutrient deficiencies," says Ellyn Satter, R.D., author of *Secrets of Feeding a Healthy Family* (Kelcy Press, Madison, Wis., 1999).

With lacto-ovo vegetarian diets (which include milk and eggs), it's relatively easy to supply all the nutrients both an adult and a growing child need, since these diets contain foods from all five food groups (vegetables, fruit, whole grains, nonfat milk, and legumes). The going gets tough with vegan diets, which exclude all animal products. These diets require careful planning or they will be low in iron, zinc, protein, calcium, iodine, and vitamins B_2, B_{12}, B_6, and D.

A vegetarian who wants to adopt the Origin Diet should eat all the same foods, with the exception that at least three servings of protein/iron-rich beans must be included in the daily diet. If you also have eliminated milk products, then make sure to include three servings (8 ounces each) daily of calcium- and vitamin-D-fortified soymilk.

Beyond Flintstones:
The Whys and Hows of Supplements

Our ancient ancestors ate pounds of Mother Nature's most nutrient-packed wild foods. Even if you followed all of the Origin dietary guidelines, you'd be hard-pressed to reach the levels of vitamins and minerals in those original diets. It's not that our soils are depleted or that conventional produce is less nutritious than organic, it's just that domesticated plants aren't as nutritionally concentrated as wild ones, our diets are not as varied, and we don't exercise enough to eat as much as our ancestors did.

Of the 40-plus essential nutrients required for optimal health, some are a breeze, while others are close to impossible to get from food alone. Today it's difficult to obtain the 1,900 milligrams of calcium, the 600 milligrams of vitamin C, or the 10,000 IU of beta carotene, to name only a few, found in those ancient diets. According to recent research, you also need daily at least 100 IU of vitamin E to lower heart disease risk and possibly improve immune response. That equates to 25 cups of blueberries, 4½ cups of wheat germ, or 2⅓ cups of olive oil every day! Frankly, I don't know where people are expected to get their vitamin D when they don't drink two to four glasses of vitamin D-fortified milk or soymilk every day, eat fortified cereal every morning, or spend time in the sun (without sunscreen lotion).

When it comes to some nutrients, supplements might be even better than food. In a study from the University of Ulster in Northern Ireland, blood levels of folic acid rose only in women who supplemented or consumed folic-acid-fortified foods, while folic acid from food didn't do the trick. People absorb vitamin K thirty-three times better from supplements than from spinach, one of the richest dietary sources of this vitamin. Seniors also absorb vitamin B_{12} better in supplement form than from foods.

That's not saying you should choose supplements over food. Most nutrients, such as iron, are much better absorbed from food (in this case from meat) than from supplements or fortified foods. Besides, fruits, vegetables, beans, whole grains, and other minimally processed foods supply more than just vitamins and minerals. They are Mother Nature's best sources of fiber and thousands of phytochemicals that you can't get from supplements. The bottom line: Follow the Origin Diet *and* supplement responsibly. Here's how.

SUPPLEMENTS 101

Where do you start? With a multiple, of course! But, even here you must separate the diamonds from the stones. Look for:

- The USP seal on the label. United States Pharmacopoeia, or USP, is a nongovernmental standard-setting body. This seal of quality means that the supplement should dissolve within the digestive tract, is made from pure ingredients, and contains the amount of nutrients listed on the label.

- A broad-range multiple that contains vitamins A, D, and K, all of the B vitamins (vitamins B_1, B_2, B_6, B_{12}, niacin, and folic acid), and the trace minerals (chromium, copper, iron, manganese, selenium, and zinc). Ignore chloride, pantothenic acid, biotin, potassium, choline, and phosphorus, since the diet either already supplies optimal levels of these compounds or supplements contain too little to be useful. Also ignore nickel, iodine, vanadium, and tin; it's not clear whether we need these minerals.

• A multiple that provides approximately 100 percent, but no more than 300 percent, of the Daily Value for all nutrients provided. You want a balanced supplement, not one that supplies 2 percent of one nutrient, 25 percent of another, and 600 percent of another.

Besides a multiple, there are three other supplements to consider. The first is a calcium-magnesium supplement. No single-dose multiple supplies enough calcium and magnesium, so consider taking a calcium-magnesium supplement if you consume less than three glasses of nonfat milk and several servings of magnesium-rich soybeans, wheat germ, and dark green leafy vegetables each day. A supplement that supplies about 500 milligrams of calcium and 250 milligrams of magnesium will fill in any nutritional gaps in your diet.

DO KIDS NEED VITAMINS?

Most kids probably need a little nutritional insurance. During the pre-teen years, children have high nutrient needs and small appetites. Young children can also be finicky eaters or eat sporadically. Even under ideal conditions, it is not always possible to get children to eat well. In a recent study from the National Cancer Institute, like adults, only one out of every one hundred kids meets the minimal standards of a balanced diet. As a result, many of our children consume less than half the recommended amount of iron and zinc. Intakes of calcium, B vitamins, vitamin C, vitamin A, vitamin E, and other essential nutrients are often low in children's diets. Also, eating well during the early years sets the stage for health in the future. For example, calcium intake in childhood is essential to building strong, dense bones resistant to osteoporosis later in life. A moderate-dose multiple vitamin and mineral supplement, plus extra calcium and magnesium, fill in the gaps on those days your child doesn't eat perfectly.

The second supplement to consider is an antioxidant. If your multiple doesn't contain extra vitamin E, consider taking a third supplement of 100 to 400 IU of this antioxidant. Finally, if you can't include at least three servings of omega-3-rich foods in your weekly diet, such as salmon or omega-3-enriched spaghetti sauce or eggs, then consider taking a daily fish oil capsule that supplies about 1 to 2 grams of docosahexaenoic acid (DHA) and/or eicosapentaenoic acid (EPA).

When should you take your supplements? The time of day is not as important as what you take them with. Most nutrients are best absorbed when taken with meals and in small doses throughout the day (the inconvenience of taking divided doses might make a one-pill-a-day product more appealing). For maximum absorption, take a multiple with iron at a different meal than your calcium supplement, since these two minerals compete for absorption.

SUPPLEMENT ECONOMICS

Supplements that cost more are not necessarily better. Supplement companies buy their raw ingredients from the same suppliers, so the vitamin C in one pill is the same as in another. In fact, if you're paying more than about ten dollars a month for any or all of your supplements, you're spending too much. You can find quality multiple vitamin and mineral supplements that cost less than ten cents a day, or three dollars a month. Add another one to three dollars a month for a good calcium-magnesium supplement, and about the same for an antioxidant or vitamin E capsule.

To cut costs, steer clear of the following:

- Extra ingredients like lipoic acid, enzymes, primrose oil, or inositol, to name only a few. These extras only add cost, but are either worthless or supplied in amounts too low to be of use.
- Time-released vitamins. There is no proof they are better absorbed than regular vitamins.
- "Natural" supplements. They're costly and usually provide no added benefit over other supplements. (Exceptions to this rule are vitamin E,

The Stone Age Supplement

Put together your own supplement program, based on the following optimal intakes, which resemble the nutrient intakes of our ancient ancestors. You should be able to meet these needs by taking two to four tablets (a multiple, antioxidants, calcium, and magnesium, or calcium-magnesium tablets) daily with meals.

NUTRIENT	OPTIMAL AMOUNT
Vitamin A (retinol)	2,500 IU
Beta carotene	15 mg
Vitamin D	400 IU
Vitamin E (D-alpha tocopherol)	200–400 IU
Vitamin B$_1$ (thiamine)	2–6 mg
Vitamin B$_2$ (riboflavin)	2–6 mg
Niacin (niacinamide)	20 mg
Vitamin B$_6$ (pyridoxine)	2–10 mg
Vitamin B$_{12}$ (cobalamin)	6–10 mcg
Folic acid (folacin)	400–600 mcg
Vitamin K	65 mcg
Pantothenic acid	10 mg
Vitamin C	250–1,000 mg
Calcium (calcium carbonate)	1,200–1,500 mg
Chromium (chromium-rich yeast, picolinate, or nicotinate)	200 mcg
Copper	2 mg
Iron (ferrous fumarate)	18 mg*
Magnesium (magnesium citrate)	500 mg
Manganese	5 mg
Molybdenum	75–250 mcg
Selenium (L-selenomethionine)	200 mcg
Zinc	15–30 mg

*Iron supplements are recommended only for women during the childbearing years. Men and postmenopausal women should take iron supplements only with approval from their physicians.

selenium, and chromium; if you can afford the added costs, these three appear to be better absorbed and used by the body in their natural form than their inorganic or synthetic forms.)

• Chelated minerals (which are chemically bound to an amino acid). Again, there is no convincing evidence that they are any better absorbed or used by the body than other minerals. The same goes for colloidal minerals.

• "Women's" or "men's" formulas. Women's nutritional needs are different from men's, so theoretically a special formula would more closely match their needs. But you'll be hard-pressed to find a good product. Most are formulated more on marketing than on science, falling far short of optimal and costing much more than well-formulated multiples. You're better off following the above guidelines than you are selecting a supplement because of its name.

When the unit price saves you money, purchase bigger or "economy size" bottles or store-brand products (they are often made by the same companies that make the brand-name supplements). Make sure you can use the supplements before the expiration date on the label to ensure potency.

6

The Origin Workout

Man still bears in his bodily frame the indelible stamp of his . . . origin.

—CHARLES DARWIN, 1871

We are meant to be fit. Our bodies thrive on physical activity. Our health depends on it. It is not merely chance that people in excellent physical condition are at low risk for disease, live longer, enjoy optimistic outlooks and good moods, handle stress well, think clearly, and look younger than their years. Exercise arouses the body, sharpens the senses, increases blood flow to the muscles and brain, increases the transportation of oxygen and nutrients to the tissues, speeds the removal of toxins and cellular debris, and reduces overall stress on the body. The reasons why exercise is so critical to our well-being date back about 5 million years.

The Five-Million-Year-Old Runner

Your body's need for activity dates back to its very origins. All of your ultra-ancient ancestors, spanning hundreds of thousands and even millions of years, thrived on vigorous activity. About 5 million years ago, our humanlike ancestors stood up and started walking on two feet, a skill achieved by no other primate. Their striding, graceful gait allowed all of our ancestors to walk and run efficiently for miles. As far back as 3.6 million years ago, our ultra-ancient ancestors were already adept at long-distance exercise, as shown by the fossilized remains of two sets of foot-prints walking side by side in the volcanic dust of what is now Laetoli, Tanzania.

We are designed for sport. Our hairless bodies allow air to flow over our skin, especially when we walk or run, which quickly dissipates heat. Humans are one of the few animals (other than horses, camels, and cattle) that sweat. This allowed our ancient ancestors to be active on the hot savanna and allows us today to work in hot weather without over-heating. Our bodies are 40 percent muscle, primed to move us long dis-tances and to lift or carry heavy loads.

Fast-forward to 40,000 years ago, when people just like us populated the world. If alive today, they would be physicians, schoolteachers, com-puter analysts, waiters, and taxi drivers. It's just that back then, their main occupation was as full-time hunters and gatherers. That job required an immense amount of physical exertion. They took to this active lifestyle like fish to water, since their heritage was one of vigorous activity. The stories their parents and grandparents told around the campfire in the evenings were of ancestors who were skilled at spear throwing, archery, wielding axes, chasing down game, or harpooning seals. They grew up on stories of how a great-uncle or great-grandfather had outrun a gazelle, which fed the tribe during a harsh winter, or of how a great-great-grandmother, with her baby strapped to her back, walked six miles back to camp carrying the largest yam found that year, weighing twenty-five pounds. These people maintained superior physical fitness to accomplish these feats, just as an Olympic athlete today trains for years before competing.

Life as a hunter-gatherer required incredible endurance, stamina, and strength. Men tracked, stalked, and pursued game for hours and even days. Women walked long distances carrying heavy loads of produce and children. They moved camp every few weeks to follow the game and food supply. They walked long distances to visit relatives and neighbors. Their leisure activities often included dancing and other vigorous activi-ties. They even burned hundreds of calories every day just keeping their bodies warm in the winter and cool in the summer. Those who were capable of high levels of physical endurance and strength were the ones who survived to pass on their genes to the next generation.

Their genes are our genes. All of us, not just professional athletes, carry within us the same potential for fitness. Modern-day hunter-gatherers remind us of this. The Tarahumara Indians in northern Mexico participate in 25- to 150-mile races lasting up to forty-eight hours and traversing rugged terrain. Ache tribesmen in Paraguay chase their prey, such as deer and wild pigs, to exhaustion. These physical skills seem heroic, much like the performance of professional dancers or Olympian athletes, yet are typical of people who live physically vigorous lives.

Hello Laptop, Good-Bye Muscles

- How much muscular exertion have you expended in the hours you've been reading this book?
- How many hours did it take to hunt down and capture your last meal?
- How many calories did you spend preparing that meal? Did it require shelling, grinding, butchering, or merely opening a box?
- How long did it take you to gather the wood or fuel to cook that meal?
- How much shivering or sweating have you done in the past week?
- How many hours of vigorous work have you done today?

If you're like most people, you have expended next to nothing in physical activity in the past few hours, live in a temperature-controlled home, and drive to the grocery store. We are the most unfit humans that have ever walked the earth. We work in swivel chairs, push powered lawn mowers, sit behind steering wheels, and use remote controls. A single phone extension "saves" the typical American about seventy miles of walking each year. As obesity expert Dr. John Foreyt says, "The obesity epidemic results from a clash between our hunter-gatherer ancient genes and our modern sedentary lifestyles."

A typical American burns daily in physical activity only 2.04 calories per pound of body weight, or about 306 calories for a 150-pound person. Compare that to modern-day hunter-gatherers, who typically burn about 11.36 calories per pound of body weight every day, or about 1,704 calories. Even our children are sedentary, sitting in classrooms during the day, then sitting in front of a television or computer in the evening. This is a far cry from Paleolithic children, who spent their days running, walking, learning to throw spears and use hand axes, climbing, and leaping. In short, our bodies evolved from being more active in one day than the typical person today is in five days.

Our sedentary lifestyles are matched only by our even more sedentary leisure activities. While walking and running were the only means of transportation up until six thousand years ago, when the horse was domesticated, today walking has become so rare that new housing developments are designed without sidewalks. The statistics are frightening:

- Only one in nine adults exercises regularly during his or her leisure time.
- Two out of five American adults are classified as downright sedentary, with heart rates seldom rising above an idle.
- Only 15 percent of adults include some form of exercise at least three times a week for twenty minutes or more.
- By age seventy-five, a third of all men and half of all women don't exercise at all.

Sedentary living seems normal to us, but it is as pathologically alien to our bodies as being bedridden. As we gave up the spear and then the plow for push-button cell phones, cars, and computers, our muscles atrophied, our body fat ballooned, and our risk for disease skyrocketed.

Exercise Away Disease

Our ultra-ancient ancestors sidestepped disease by staying fit. Like them, our health also depends on staying physically active. Hundreds of studies show that people who are physically fit are healthier than sedentary couch potatoes. Compared to inactive people, a person who exercises daily has lower blood pressure, lower blood cholesterol, higher HDL cholesterol (the "good" cholesterol), and has as much as a 40 percent lower risk of developing heart disease, and an even lower risk of dying from it. For example:

- A study from the Harvard School of Public Health found that the risk of dying prematurely from any cause decreased as people increased their participation in vigorous activity.
- A study from the Cooper Institute for Aerobic Research found that unfit men were as likely to die as men who had suffered a heart attack or stroke. Steven Blair, Ph.D., lead researcher of the study, was "surprised to see that low fitness was actually a stronger predictor of mortality than was diabetes, high blood pressure, high cholesterol, or current smoking."
- A joint statement from the American College of Sports Medicine and the Centers for Disease Control and Prevention in Atlanta estimates that 250,000 deaths each year in the United States can be attributed to physical inactivity alone. That staggering figure places lethargy in the same high-risk category as smoking, obesity, hypertension, and drunk driving.

Physically active people, compared to exercise avoiders, are leaner and have better insulin sensitivity, thus lowering their risk of high blood pressure and diabetes. (Up to 44 percent of deaths in people who are overweight could be prevented by exercise, compared to 9 percent of deaths if diabetes was prevented!) Compared to sedentary people, exercisers are less likely to develop colon cancer, stroke, or back injuries. They have stronger bones more resistant to osteoporosis, and they are up to 25 percent less likely to injure themselves or even fall compared to unfit people.

It's also astounding how quickly the body responds to exercise. Years ago I worked at a medically based program for people with advanced heart disease, diabetes, and high blood pressure. Most patients faced open-heart surgery or death as their only other options. Yet within two weeks of eating well and exercising daily under the supervision of a physician and exercise physiologist, patients who had been unable to walk the length of the hospital hallway on entry into the program were walking briskly on treadmills with smiles on their faces! Blood cholesterol levels dropped 20 percent, triglycerides fell even further, and patients who had entered the program on up to eleven different medications left on fewer or no medications.

The Anti-Aging Effect

Sitting on your duff won't do you in when you're fifteen, twenty, or even twenty-five years old. But by your thirties, your muscles are already starting to weaken. We lose approximately 1 to 2 percent of muscle mass every year after this point, which equates to a five-to-ten pound loss of muscle every decade. You don't notice the lost muscle until you're in your forties, when pushing a door open takes two hands instead of one or you unconsciously take the elevator to avoid the stairs.

As the aging body loses muscle, it accumulates fat. Fat is inactive tissue, requiring few calories to maintain. The more fat you have, the fewer calories you need to maintain a constant body weight. In contrast, the muscular bodies of our ancient ancestors were metabolic hotbeds of activity, burning fuel or calories when moving and even when at rest. It's no wonder that both Paleolithic evidence as well as studies on modern-day hunter-gatherers show that people living in tune with their bodies stay lean, strong, and vital no matter what their ages.

The fat-for-muscle trade-off is alien to our bodies and results in the general body breakdown we associate with aging. First, our metabolic rate plummets. It takes fewer calories to keep going, so you'll gain weight at forty-five years old if you eat like a twenty-year-old. The gradual loss of muscle leads to the opposite of the Paleolithic robust vitality inherent in our bodies. We become weak and sluggish, which further slows our activity level. As our muscle slips away, we age more rapidly. Our bones become porous without the constant tug of muscles to keep them strong. The accumulation of body fat around our middles leads to increased blood cholesterol and glucose, elevated blood pressure, and increased insulin resistance, which place us at increased risk for most age-related illnesses, from heart disease and diabetes to hypertension and cancer. Silently and gradually it takes more effort to do even simple daily tasks; consequently, you do less and less. If you live long enough, you'll reach a point where you can't get out of a chair without help, cross the street without feeling winded, or even pick up the groceries, let alone your grandchild.

The good news is that none of this decline is necessary; it certainly isn't normal. Anyone, no matter what his or her age, who begins exercis-

STILL NOT CONVINCED?

Our bodies must move to stay healthy. It's not so much that exercise decreases our risk for disease as that not exercising causes our bodies to deteriorate. If you exercise daily, you can expect to:

- Decrease your risk of developing or dying from heart disease.
- Prevent or delay the development of high blood pressure.
- Decrease your blood pressure.
- Lower your risk of developing non-insulin-dependent diabetes.
- Lower your risk of developing cancer.
- Maintain youthful muscle strength.
- Improve the range of motion, structure, and function of your joints, reducing your risk for developing arthritis and lessening its pain and stiffness.
- Control joint swelling associated with arthritis.
- Attain peak bone mass.
- Slow bone loss associated with aging, thus reducing your risk of developing osteoporosis.
- Reduce the likelihood of gaining excess body fat and have an easier time losing excess body fat.
- Increase your lean body mass.

- Improve your digestive function.
- Improve your lung and respiratory function.
- Have an easier time adopting other healthful habits.
- Improve your sleep pattern.
- More easily perform daily tasks.
- Have more energy and less fatigue.
- Reduce your risk for depression, anxiety, and stress.
- Feel better, happier, and more positive.
- Boost your self-esteem and self-confidence.
- Better regulate your appetite, with fewer cravings and less overeating.
- Age gracefully with less chance of losing your independence.
- Look ten to twenty years younger.
- Reduce your risk of falling.
- Maintain a revved metabolic rate.
- Recover more quickly from illness.

ing shows increases in muscle and improvements in strength and meta-bolic rates. People who continue to exercise in their second fifty years are as fit or even fitter than sedentary women who are twenty to thirty years younger, which might explain why they also live longer. Middle-aged men who take up exercise lower their risk of dying prematurely by a third. In fact, there's an inverse relationship between physical activity and longevity; the more calories people expend in exercise each week the longer they are likely to live free of disease. All you must do is keep moving in tune with your evolutionary heritage. By staying fit and strong like you were meant to be, you can rewrite your script for health, energy, and aging at almost any age.

Vital Movement

Watch the faces on the people out for a brisk walk or feel the enthusi-asm of bicyclists lined up for a race. Listen to people at your local gym.

In all cases, you hear and see the signs of optimism, exuberance, enthu- siasm, and encouragement. Our bodies need daily physical activity, like they need sleep and nutritious food. Exercise empowers us, refreshes our minds, and keeps us vibrant.

Our moods depend as much on our activity levels as do our hearts and bones. A daily workout releases brain chemicals, such as epinephrine and norepinephrine, which boost alertness. Regular exercise also raises levels of serotonin, a nerve chemical that boosts mood in much the same way as antidepressants like Prozac. Daily activity naturally de-stresses the body by lowering blood levels of the stress hormones, including cortisol, that prepare the body for "fight or flight." In addition, the rise in body temperature that results from a vigorous workout has a tranquilizing effect on the body, not unlike soaking in a hot tub.

Then, of course, there's the "exercise high," that burst of euphoria that follows vigorous activity. This natural high is probably caused by the release of endorphins, the body's natural morphine-like chemicals that help boost pain tolerance and generate feelings of euphoria and satisfac- tion. "Exercise is one of the best remedies for depression, sometimes better even than medications or counseling," says Ed Pierce, Ph.D., asso- ciate professor in the Department of Health and Sport Science at the University of Richmond in Virginia.

Throughout their lives, physically fit people are happier, more satis- fied with their lives, and less prone to depression, anxiety, and stress than people who don't exercise. Active people also think more clearly, con- centrate better, remember more, and react quicker than sedentary folks—obvious benefits in the more severe days of our ancestors and critical to a quality life today.

Maybe it's not that exercise is an antidepressant, but rather that *not* exercising is so abnormal to our bodies that it leads to emotional deterioration. In one study, researchers compared the effects of no exer- cise versus various intensities of exercise on psychological outcomes. After twelve months, the sedentary subjects were the ones battling the most stress, anxiety, and depression, while the exercisers felt great. Our bodies are grateful for any type of activity, so both endurance activities, such as walking, running, or swimming, and strength training alleviate depression and improve mood.

In short, physically fit bodies allow us the freedom to do what we want and the energy to fuel our motivation to participate fully in life and to enjoy every minute of it. Opting to be sedentary is the riskiest vice you can choose. Ironically, those people who stick with an exercise program for at least six months report that if only they'd known how good they would feel, they would have started exercising earlier! And it's as simple as getting off the couch and moving—every day for the rest of your life—just like the billions of ancestors before you.

Stone Age Secret #1:
Stay Strong and Lean

> Everyone is an athlete. The only difference is that some of us are in training, and some are not.
>
> —GEORGE SHEEHAN, M.D.

To put it simply, to regain control of your true nature, you must live a vigorously active life. The more you move, the better you'll feel, the more energy you'll have, the less you'll fall victim to daily health problems or serious disease down the road, the longer you'll live, and the more you'll enjoy the extra years. To reap these rewards only takes daily exercise and adding more activity to your daily routine.

Whether you are young and injury-free, a senior with creaky joints, physically challenged, or exercise phobic, you can find an activity routine that works for you. Here's how to incorporate this secret into your daily life.

JUST DO IT—RIGHT

We were born to cross-train. Our bodies evolved on vigorous activity that varied from one day to the next. That means we must vary our sport from day to day, rather than only take an aerobic dance class or only bicycle. To do this exercise thing right means moving as your body evolved to move by cycling activities between

1. a variety of endurance activities, such as walking, rowing, swimming, or jogging;
2. a variety of strength training activities, such as lifting weights or calisthenics like sit-ups;
3. flexibility exercises; and
4. rest.

How Many Minutes Does It Take to Burn the 150 Calories in a Small Doughnut?

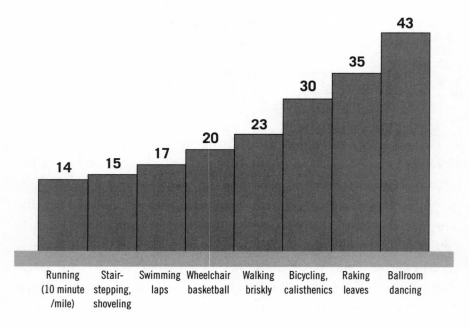

Running (10 minute /mile)	Stair-stepping, shoveling	Swimming laps	Wheelchair basketball	Walking briskly	Bicycling, calisthenics	Raking leaves	Ballroom dancing
14	15	17	20	23	30	35	43

The endurance activity strengthens your heart and keeps you lean, while strength training builds muscles and boosts your metabolic rate. Flexibility activities allow your joints and muscles to move easily. Rest allows your muscles time to recuperate and build new tissue. The sooner you start, the better, but it's never too late to slow the loss and even reverse the damage.

HOW TO START

Consider the following before beginning any exercise routine:

- *Get clearance.* If you are more than forty years old, obtain clearance from your physician before beginning an exercise program. You'll need to complete a monitored fitness test, which will help you identify where you need to focus your fitness efforts, such as increasing your cardiovascular fitness level and upper body strength. Or maybe balance and flexibility are a high priority. Your physician can also help you decide at what level you should start a fitness program and if there are any undetected health risks that should be considered, such as high cholesterol or blood pressure.

- *Have a plan.* After a thorough physical evaluation, you and your physician or an exercise physiologist can map out an initial plan of action. You wouldn't set out on a vacation without knowing where you want to go and what you want to do. Yet many people jump into exercise, join a fitness club, or purchase home-exercise equipment without first sitting down and thinking it through. Even if it's something as simple as walking to work, you need to decide how you'll carry your papers or lunch, how you'll keep your work clothes clean, and even what route you'll take. You'll also need to purchase quality exercise gear.

- *Anticipate stumbling blocks.* Excuses, travel, or weather that keeps you from your normal routine can undermine the best of intentions. Write down all your personal reasons why you can't exercise, such as not enough time, can't afford it, could never lose weight, don't like to sweat, an unsupportive spouse, or it's boring. Next to each, list the reasons why that excuse isn't good enough. Remember the saying "Problems aren't barriers, only obstacles to be hurdled."

- *Make it a priority.* Exercise will become a habit only if it's at the top of your priority list. Before you book anything else into your weekly calendar, set aside a time or place five to six days a week for exercise and don't allow anyone or anything to get in the way. Expect to exercise by bringing exercise clothes with you, even when you travel. Put on your exercise clothes when you get up in the morning or when you arrive home after work; keep them on until you've exercised. You don't need huge amounts of time to exercise. You can even break your activity sessions into several mini-exercise sessions throughout the day. Research shows that you derive the same benefits from one session or two to three mini-workouts, as long as the total day's time is at least thirty minutes in the beginning and one hour as you become a seasoned exerciser.

• *Set realistic goals.* Vigorous activity is your ultimate goal, but if you haven't exercised in years, you're better off starting slow. That way you're likely to stick with it and do it longer than someone who bursts onto the exercise scene with a vengeance. Begin by stretching, walking, and doing low-weight strength training. Slowly increase the length of your workouts and their intensity. A rule of thumb is to increase the intensity of your workouts by no more than 10 percent each week to reduce the chance of injury. To see benefits, you must move enough to sweat, but not so much that soreness or fatigue nix your motivation to stick with it. Here's ways to increase your workouts safely and gradually:

- If you now walk five miles a week, increase that to five and a half miles next week, then to six miles the week after.
- If you walk three days a week, increase that to four days. Add a day roughly every two weeks until you're walking nearly every day.
- Add five minutes to your daily routine until you're walking at least three miles at a time.
- Walk at your normal pace for one minute, then extra briskly for one minute, then back to your normal pace, and so on.

• *Define how fit you want to be.* You can't do minimal amounts of exercise and expect fantastic results. Be honest with yourself when matching how much you're willing to move with the weight loss or health benefits you expect. If you don't like pain or sweat, then set a moderate pace, but realize that this routine will take more time; you'll need to gradually increase the length of your workouts to at least ninety minutes a day if you want to lose weight. If you want to save time and shave inches off your waistline, then train harder. The least you'll need to do is thirty minutes of intense endurance activity, four days a week, plus two twenty-minute strength training sessions.

VIGOROUS LIVING

> Origin recommendation: Include at least 2 hours a day of activity other than exercise.
>
> What is vigorous living? Take the stairs, park far from the store and walk, garden on the weekends, use a push lawn mower, etc.

While we think of exercise as activity separate from our daily life and usually done on leisure time, for hunter-gatherers, exercise *is* their active lives. According to recent studies from the University of Pennsylvania School of Medicine in Philadelphia and the Cooper Institute for Aerobic Research in Dallas, you benefit as much from increasing your daily activity, like taking the stairs instead of the elevator or walking instead of driving short distances, as you do from a structured exercise program. In the Pennsylvania study, overweight women either took aerobics classes for up to forty-five minutes three days a week (totaling about 1,500 calories per week of exercise) or they accumulated thirty minutes daily of moderate-intensity physical activity within their normal daily routines.

The results were astonishing! Women who increased their lifestyle activity lost about the same amount of weight compared to the women who followed a traditional aerobic exercise program. The more they moved during the day, the greater the benefits. "Compared to the exercisers, the women who increased their lifestyle activity had a greater tendency to maintain their weight loss because they continued to stay more active, while many of the exercisers dropped out of the aerobics class," says Dr. Thomas Wadden, one of the study's investigators.

How did the women boost their daily activity? According to Dr. Wadden, they stopped using their kids as servants, took mini-walks of one to five minutes several times during the day, and threw out the television remote control. Some went to the bathroom on a different floor at work (using the stairs, not the elevator to get there) or got up to talk to their coworkers rather than e-mailing them. "Ultimately, weight loss is about calories in and calories out, and you can package those calories out as either high-intensity workouts or moderate-intensity activity distributed throughout the day," says Dr. Wadden.

It Adds Up

One way to look at exercise is to monitor the number of calories you burn each week in physical exertion—including both structured exercise and everyday physical activity. If you consciously increase your walking, stair climbing, and movement throughout the day, you'll be surprised how many calories you'll burn!

ACTIVITY	CALORIES BURNED/DAY
Monday	
Walk at lunch, 30 minutes	
Climb stairs at work, 10 minutes	
Stationary bicycle while watching TV in evening, 20 minutes	252
Tuesday	
Walk at lunch, 30 minutes	
Climb stairs at work, 10 minutes	
Strength training, 25 minutes	272
Wednesday	
Walk at lunch, 30 minutes	
Climb stairs at work, 10 minutes	
Stationary bicycle while watching TV in evening, 20 minutes	252
Thursday	
Walk at lunch, 30 minutes	
Climb stairs at work, 10 minutes	
Strength training, 25 minutes	272
Friday	
Walk at lunch, 30 minutes	
Climb stairs at work, 10 minutes	140

ACTIVITY	CALORIES BURNED/DAY
Saturday	
Walk in countryside, 1 hour	
Strength training, 25 minutes	
Wash car and windows, 1 hour	523
Sunday	
Housework, 1 hour	
Gardening, 1 hour	443
Total Week:	
Hours of activity: 9 hours 15 minutes	2,154 calories!

PALEOLITHIC PLAY

Play is as natural to our health as breathing. Playfulness and spontaneity are so necessary for health that their absence is a sign of mental illness. Play reduces stress and anxiety, is an outlet for fantasy, and stimulates our brain and nervous system. People deprived of the opportunity to move and play experience hallucinations, delusions, distortions of body image, and mental dysfunction.

We might give up the doll houses and imaginary battle games as we grow up, but play is just as critical to our health as it was in our youth. Exercise is the perfect outlet for that spontaneous activity. Make exercise fun! Physical activity should bring out the kid in you. It should be your playtime during the day, where you laugh, enjoy the company of friends, and find joy in what your body can do. Doing something physical should be pleasurable, active, freeing, and rewarding.

- Listen to music or books on tape while walking.
- Explore the countryside on a bicycle.
- Explore a new city with a brisk walk.
- Sign up for charity walk-a-thons.

- Do circuit training at a playground: swing on the swings, climb the jungle gym, and ride the see-saw.
- Invite your friends over for an exercise party. Play tag on bicycles, organize a softball or basketball game, compete in relay races, or go for a hike.
- Try one new sport each month.

Eventually, exercise can become something you'd do even if it had no benefits other than the inherent joy in doing it.

That might mean linking efforts with friends if you are a social animal or choosing a solitary sport if you need quiet time away from the rat race. It might mean alternating three or more activities throughout the week to keep your exercise-play fresh and new. Most important is that you'll stick with exercise only if it's fun. So ask yourself what you like to do and what is realistic to do, then use your imagination to keep exercise interesting.

Boost Endurance

Origin recommendation: At first, a daily total of twenty minutes, five days a week. Ultimate goal is forty-five to sixty minutes, five days a week.

What is an endurance sport? Anything that gets your heart pumping, including aerobic dance, step aerobics, bicycling, stationary cycling, hiking, jumping rope, rowing, running/jogging, stair climbing, skating, cross-country skiing, snowshoeing, StairMaster machine, swimming, trampolining, brisk walking (4-plus miles per hour).

Our bodies need to rove, walk, saunter, and run. Our hearts depend on this form of endurance activity for cardiovascular fitness. Our blood vessels and blood pressure need long-distance activity to keep them in working order. Our muscles and tissues thrive only when they're supplied with the flood of oxygen provided by long-distance activity.

The plus side is that endurance activities burn more calories and body fat than any other activity. Most bodies can't maintain a desirable weight without it. Another advantage of a long walk is that it tempers the stress response by lowering stress hormone levels and raising brain levels of endorphins, which calms us and leaves us feeling refreshed and happy. Endurance activity also lowers our risk for developing elevated blood cholesterol and heart disease.

If you've been sedentary, then some activity is better than none; if you're already active, then more exercise is better than some. The guidelines for the endurance portion of your exercise program are easy. Just make sure to:

1. Warm up for five to ten minutes before beginning the activity.
2. Include movements that are continual and rhythmic, and that use the major muscle groups, such as the arms and legs.
3. Pay attention to your heart rate and perceived exertion level during the activity.
4. Keep within your target heart rate (see below and the box on page 188).
5. Vary the sport. For example, walk one day and bicycle the next.
6. Make it fun, playful, and enjoyable.
7. Build up to at least forty-five minutes of continuous motion.
8. Cool down for five to ten minutes after the activity, including some stretching and flexibility exercises.

A basic guideline is to exercise at a level that allows you to talk and sweat at the same time. If you can't talk, you're exercising too hard and should slow down, even if you're within your target heart rate (THR). If you are within your THR and can sing or whistle while exercising, you are not working hard enough, so you should increase your exertion to the higher end of the THR scale.

Build Strength

Origin recommendation: Include at least two, preferably four, strength training sessions in your weekly routine. Change the routine by varying the combination of sets, repetitions, weights, and resistance.

YOUR TARGET HEART RATE

1. Identify your maximum heart rate (MHR) by subtracting your age from 220.

2. Identify your target heart rate (THR) by multiplying your MHR by 0.60 to 0.90. For example, a forty-year-old person's THR would be:

   220 − 40 = 180 (MHR)

   180 (MHR) × 0.60=108 beats per minute for 60 percent of MHR

   180 (MHR) × 0.90=162 beats per minute for 90 percent of MHR

   This person's THR is between 108 and 162 beats per minute.

3. Monitor your heart rate during exercise by lightly placing your two middle fingers on your throat, just to the side of center. Don't press too hard or you'll slow the pulse. Or, place two fingers on the thumb side of your wrist. In either case, start with zero on the first beat and count for ten seconds. Then multiply that number by six, or count for six seconds and add a zero to the end of that figure to obtain the total heart beats per one minute. It is important to count the pulse immediately after stopping exercise, since the pulse rate slows quickly once exercise is stopped.

When our ancestors weren't walking and running, they were lifting, digging, hauling, and pushing. While endurance activities will pamper your heart, strength training will keep you young. Both help you maintain a healthy weight. You can't just walk and assume you're doing enough. Even highly trained runners suffer from weakened muscles, nagging injuries, and increasing weight gain as they age, unless they combine their endurance workouts with at least two strength training sessions weekly.

Strength training preserves and restores muscle tissue. The added muscle shifts metabolism into high gear with an increased calorie burn of about 7.5 percent for up to fifteen hours after the workout. Unless you combine endurance activity with strength training when trying to lose weight, you'll lose lean tissue and end up weaker from dieting.

The natural strength training of modern-day hunter-gatherers pre-vents the muscle and joint injuries that we associate with aging. An added benefit is that strong muscles allow you to perform daily tasks with less effort, so you accomplish more and have energy left over! Strengthening and flexibility exercises for the abdominal, pelvic, and spinal muscles also improve posture, which helps coordination, balance, and range of motion.

Lifting weights doesn't mean you'll bulk up like a bodybuilder. It does firm your body, help you drop a pants size or two (muscle is denser than fat so your body measurements drop even if the pounds on the scale don't show the fat loss), and prevent needless aches and pains. It also revs metabolism.

You can do well-designed calisthenics at home, adding hand and ankle weights as you progress. Or purchase free weights or machines to use at home or join the gym. When you meet with a trained exercise physiologist or fitness expert to determine the best muscle-building pro-gram for you, make sure you:

1. Include exercises that strengthen the muscles at the back of the thigh (hamstrings), front thigh (quadriceps), lower back (erector spinae), abdominals, chest (pectorals), upper back, upper arms (biceps and triceps), shoulders, and neck.
2. Include warm-up and cool-down exercises before and after strength training.
3. Work each muscle group to near fatigue, or about one to three sets of eight to twelve repetitions each. Choose weights that are heavy enough that you can't do any more than twelve repetitions at a time. At first, it might take only lifting the weight equivalent of a jug of milk or a hardbound dictionary. When the last few lifts are too easy, it's time to switch to slightly heavier weights or add another set.
4. Gradually add more weight or repetitions. Don't push it. If you start with eight repetitions of fifteen pounds, you might increase to

twelve repetitions at the same weight, then increase to two sets at eight repetitions, and so forth. People often make the mistake of adding too much weight or too many repetitions too quickly, which sets them up for injury and discouragement.

5. Don't hold your breath. Inhale before you lift and exhale as you lift a weight.

6. Give your body at least one day off between sessions, or alternate upper body and lower body workouts every other day. Either option allows muscles to heal and maximizes strength gains.

Stay Flexible

Origin recommendation: Stretch for five to ten minutes before and after every endurance and strength-training workout.

Injuries, stiff joints, and muscle spasms are not signs of age, they are signs that your body has lost flexibility. By the third decade of life, subtle changes in muscle and connective tissues cause joints, ligaments, tendons, and other tissues to become increasingly more stiff and less functional, which makes us prone to injury. But older folks in hunter-gatherer societies are just as limber as the young, so this stiffening is not a decree. You must be willing to spend a few minutes every day stretching. Just remember:

1. Stretch slowly.
2. Don't bounce.
3. Don't stretch to the point of pain.
4. Breathe.

How do you know if you've warmed up sufficiently? The body temperature rises with good warm-up exercises. You've sufficiently warmed up when you break into a mild sweat. Consult your physician or physical therapist when designing a safe and effective stretching program, especially if you are recovering from any injury.

Take a Day Off

Origin recommendation: One to two days every week, go for a walk or do some mild activity different from your normal routine.

What does it mean to rest? Stroll through the countryside, walk the mall, play a game of badminton with the kids, do some light gardening, go for a leisurely bike ride, go ballroom dancing with your spouse.

Life was not all work and no play for our ancestors. Our bodies evolved on a weekly diet of about nineteen hours of vigorous activity laced with lots of sitting around the campfire telling stories, making spear points, and painting cave walls. Compensatory quiet time after intense physical activity is a natural cycle for all animals. (Does your dog flop on the kitchen floor after a long walk? Does your cat take a nap after a raucous play session?) That's probably why researchers find today that muscles heal and build better when given a day off from exercise.

This doesn't mean you should sleep all day. Take this opportunity to do some fun outdoor activity with the kids, clean the house, or plant flowers. Our need for fresh air and the great outdoors will be discussed in detail in the next chapter.

Stick With It

You make a New Year's resolution to exercise more. You start taking a spin-cycling class three times a week. By the fourth week, you're making it to class once a week, and by the second month the gym bag is at the back of the hall closet.

Our ancestors didn't have a choice. They either moved or died. Today, just knowing we should exercise isn't enough to get and keep most of us motivated to stick with it for life. There must be an immediate reward to keep moving toward the long-term hope of feeling great. It could take your body six weeks before daily exercise feels even slightly good. How are you going to motivate yourself to stick with it? How will you avoid being part of the statistic that shows most people burn out within six months of starting an exercise program?

Embracing any habit requires a full-on commitment, both in attitude and actions. Toss the old vision of yourself as inactive and start visualizing and defining yourself as an exerciser. Look for excuses to exercise, rather than reasons why you can't. Hang out with people at work, church, and in the neighborhood who exercise in their free time. Join a gym. Read exercise books, subscribe to health magazines, rent exercise or fitness tapes, take a volleyball class from the parks and recreation department in your city, and talk about exercise with other enthusiasts. For one week, keep an hourly log of how often you sit and sleep. Some people who have adopted the Origin Diet and exercise program comment that seeing on paper how much of their days is inactive was enough to get them moving! Your attitude probably won't shift overnight, but gradually you'll notice a transformation as you move from slouch to mover to avid exerciser.

Create a motivation plan. This could be something as simple as putting stars on a calendar every day that you exercise; a month of stars entitles you to a movie or a trip to the beach. Use an exercise log to plan your weekly exercise and to mark how closely you accomplished your goals. (See the activity log on page 193.) Place a dollar in a jar every day you exercise, then use the money to buy something you've always wanted. Reward yourself whenever you reach a fitness goal by purchasing clothes in your new smaller size, joining a health club, or taking a fitness-oriented vacation.

If you are a social person, then use exercise as your time to visit with friends. Take your lunch hour to walk with coworkers or friends, then grab a light snack afterward. Do you want more time with your spouse? Use exercise as a daily getaway to visit and share positive time. (One in every two people who stick with an exercise program do so because of family and social support.)

Pay attention to subtle rewards. Since you've been exercising, do you notice you have more energy? More tolerance? Feel less stressed? Sleep better? Enjoy relationships more? How is life different when you feel

THE ACTIVITY LOG

Write down your activity to keep yourself on track. Copy this page to record your daily and weekly activity. Write down your long-term and week's goals, and how you will reward yourself if, *and only if*, you meet your goals.

Week/Dates: _____

Long-Term Activity Goal: _____

This Week's Activity Goal: _____

My reward for meeting this weekly goal will be: _____

Date/Day	Activity Strength Training/ Endurance	Time	Intensity*	How Felt Afterward	Other Payoffs[†]
Weekly Wrap-Up:					

Goals (circle one):   Met   Exceeded   Not quite   Not even close

If not, what got in the way and how will I overcome that barrier next week?

_____

Exercise notes: _____

*Intensity: 1=mild, 2=moderate (broke a sweat), 3=high
[†]Improvements in sleep patterns, energy level, general well-being, ability to concentrate or think, tolerance, stress level, relationships, outlook, humor, etc.

vigorous and good? Maybe it's something as simple as forgiving the woman who cut in front of you in line or having more stamina to solve a problem at work. Write down the benefits as you notice them and tally the results each week. Use the activity log to keep track of your goals and rewards.

The Biggest Reward of All

You don't need to work out for nineteen hours a week like your Paleolithic ancestors. You just need to *move* more. Keep your body in motion for at least twenty minutes if you're a beginner and forty-five to sixty minutes if you're an avid exerciser. If the thought of target heart rates and lifting weights seems daunting, then forget all of that for now. Just move every day, with the plan that you'll move a little more every week. Your ultimate goal is to build your stamina, endurance, and strength to the point where you are vigorously active five days a week. I guarantee it will be the best gift you've ever given to yourself, both today and in the future. As Dr. George Sheehan said, "There is no substitute for learning to live in our bodies. All the tests and all the machines in the world will fail if we do not first become good animals."

7

Your Natural Rhythms

The sun was setting over the savanna as the men returned from a three-day hunting trip. The women and children met them with open arms, cheers, and praise. Hugs were laced with tears of relief that beloved friends and family members had returned safely. It was obvious the hunt had been successful, but at a cost. One young man with a serious leg wound had been carried back to camp. An elder told of an attack by a lioness. Yet they were home, and with enough meat to feed the clan for a week. The next few days would be filled with stories of the hunt and all the festivities, rest, and socializing that accompanied good times.

Our bodies evolved on more than just certain types of food and amounts of activity. Sealed into our genes millions of years ago are the origins of how we handle stress, why we must balance exercise with rest, the importance of feeling part of a community, and why immersing ourselves in nature is as important to our health as it is to our souls.

Many of us can't go back to living in small groups and few wish to live outdoors in caves, but we can re-create some of our heritage in our modern lives. We reduce our risk of disease, think more clearly, live longer, and find more satisfaction in life when we live in harmony with our ancient legacy by coping with stress as our ancestors did, enjoying quiet time to reflect, nurturing close relationships, and spending time in our original home—the great outdoors.

Thank Heaven for Stress!

The young lad attacked by the lioness was saved from being dinner because of his stress response. He first heard a branch break somewhere behind him. His mind instantly analyzed the situation: Was it a lion or the wind? How far away was the sound? Where were the others? What was the likelihood of a lion in this part of the savanna? Should he run or not? What would happen if he ran, or if he didn't? His body instantly prepared to run or fight. He felt his muscles tense, his heart race, and his breathing increase. His hearing and sense of smell became more acute. He hadn't realized his eyes had dilated to let in more light, or that inside his body a center in his brain called the hypothalamus had instantly triggered the release of the stress hormones, revving blood pressure and heart rate in preparation for action. High-octane fat fragments and quick-energy glucose had been released into his bloodstream. That oxygen-rich blood was shunted from the internal organs and skin to the muscles, heart, and brain. Arteries constricted so he'd be less likely to bleed to death if he was bitten. Within a fraction of a second he had assessed the situation and was running for his life. The lioness gave him a good swat on the leg, but his quick analysis and sprint to the nearest tree meant he lived to tell the tale.

Our response to any stressful situation, called the fight-or-flight response, ensures that our bodies automatically and instantly mount a defense against any life-threatening event by either running or fighting. The purpose of our stress response is to prepare us for danger, be it real or imagined. It was an essential response in the days when survival was threatened by attacks from saber-toothed tigers, falling off steep cliffs, being killed by a stampede, or being buried by a volcanic eruption. Many of those fears are hardwired into our bodies, which explains why children are instinctively afraid of snakes, heights, lightning, storms, loud noises, strangers, darkness, or separation. Rarely are children born with a fear of flowers, shallow water, trees, or other harmless objects from our ancient past. We've not had time to evolve innate fears of modern-day inventions, such as cigarettes, alcohol, or cars, even though they are more dangerous than snakes.

FIGHT, FLIGHT, OR STEW?

The stress response is designed for quick, effective handling of occasional threats. Immediately use those stress hormones by fighting or running and the system returns to its normal balance.

In our modern world, however, we interpret too many relatively insignificant events as life-threatening, and instead of running or fighting to discharge the stress chemicals, we sit and stew in our own juices. An endless stream of daily duties—from deadlines, traffic jams, arguments with a spouse or boss, and due dates to time pressures, mortgages, sick children, and to-do lists—causes us stress, which then lingers day in and day out, month after month. Our bodies never evolved mechanisms to handle this type of chronic stress. Consequently, normal arousal escalates into anxiety, vigilance causes insomnia, elevated heart rate and blood pressure lead to heart disease, and prolonged focused attention burns out brain cells, resulting in memory loss and learning problems.

THE COST TO OUR HEALTH

People who handle stress in a manner similar to our ancestors, by responding quickly and effectively, also are the healthiest, with low risks for physical and emotional problems, improved immunity against disease and infection, and clear thinking. Chronic stress is foreign to our bodies, upsetting the delicate checks and balances, called homeostasis, that keep us healthy. Physicians estimate that up to 75 percent of the illnesses they see are stress related. How does stewing in our own juices lead to disease?

- The liver dumps fat fragments (called fatty acids) and cholesterol into the blood, raising levels of harmful low-density lipoproteins (LDLs) and increasing the risk for heart disease.

• The constant barrage of stress hormones damages the heart muscle. One set of stress hormones, the catecholamines, alone destroys heart cells by the thousands each minute.

• The stress hormones raise the heart rate, resulting in arrhythmias (irregular heartbeat).

• Blood vessels narrow, causing high blood pressure.

• Arteries clog as they become bruised and hardened, reducing oxygen flow to the heart and increasing the risk for heart attacks.

• Contracted muscles cause back pain, headaches, and muscle spasms.

• Regions of the brain are slowly destroyed, probably by reduced blood flow and surges in cortisol. The hippocampus, the area involved in memory and emotional responses, is especially vulnerable. The brain has a limited capacity to repair damage, so as brain function is jeopardized, other tissues are affected, such as the endocrine system and nerve tissue.

• The reproductive system shuts down as body processes stay jammed in survival mode. Cortisol lowers the male hormone testosterone in men and upsets the menstrual cycle and reduces fertility in women.

• Tissues and organs not involved in survival are cut off from blood supply, which contributes to hair loss, dandruff, eczema and other skin changes, fatigue, ulcers, colitis, hyperthyroidism, kidney disease, and cold and clammy hands.

• The stress hormones raise blood glucose levels. The excess sugar attaches to proteins to form molecules called glycosylated proteins, which alter enzymes, interfere with metabolism, and increase the risk for disease. For example, glycosylated hemoglobin in red blood cells increases the risk for atherosclerosis, heart attacks, strokes, cataracts, and loss of elasticity of the arteries, joints, and lungs. These toxins also increase the risk for diabetes and premature aging.

• The stress hormone cortisol stimulates fat tissue formation and the accumulation of fat in fat cells, thus increasing the risk for obesity.

• Stress accelerates vitamin and mineral deficiencies, including calcium, magnesium, zinc, iron, copper, selenium, vitamin B_6, and the antioxidants such as vitamin C. In turn, we often make terrible food choices when we're stressed, eating too much sugar and fat (the nutrients most alien to our bodies), which aggravate the stress response, and not enough health-enhancing fruits, vegetables, and other wholesome foods.

• Stress suppresses the immune system and kills disease-fighting immune cells, leaving your body defenseless against colds, infections, asthma, arthritis, allergies, hives and rashes, and other diseases. Stressed people also take up to nine days longer to heal from cuts, scrapes, or surgery.

• Stress also affects us emotionally, increasing our risk for overeating, alcohol and drug abuse, smoking, and other self-destructive behaviors.

Bet you never realized how much damage to your body, mind, and spirit is caused by worrying! Next time you find yourself tensing behind the wheel, wound up in a knot over a deadline, or fretting that the bills won't get paid, reread the above list. Is the stress really worth losing quality time with your family? Is it worth heart disease? Is it worth losing your passion for living? Is it worth sacrificing precious years of your already limited time on earth? Is it worth dying for? Besides, most of what we worry about never even happens! It's in the best interest of your peace of mind, your arteries, your good looks, and your longevity to avoid unnecessary stress and to effectively handle the stress you can't avoid.

Our lives today are as alien to our Paleolithic bodies as living on Mars. Our tribe is now the world, not a small band of intimates. We are faced with enormous and complex societies, and venture into congested cities, not the open savanna. To override these new stressors, we must consciously use the stress response to our advantage. Learn to worry only about life-threatening stuff, and even then, react quickly and efficiently so you return to the relaxed state that restores health. Granted, everyone gets mad, worries about finances, is overwhelmed by responsibilities, and feels out of control when it comes to time. The trick is to get over it.

COPE INSTINCTIVELY WITH STRESS
A little stress is healthy. Challenges are opportunities for triumph, learning, and growth. But sometimes it's a thin line between the level of stress

that encourages us to excel and too much stress that slowly kills us. Each of us must find that balance.

Most stress is self-inflicted. We decide how busy we want to be. We choose whether or not we get angry or sad. We decide what is important in our lives. The solution to stress is different for everyone; however, the first step is recognizing that you control your life and you choose what will be stressful. In a Stone Age nutshell, to use the stress response to your advantage, you must take the following seven actions:

1. Take responsibility.

Stress is your reaction to a situation, not the situation itself. Stress doesn't happen to you. You aren't a victim. How you choose to respond to anything potentially upsetting is entirely up to you.

Granted, you have no control over the drunk driver who speeds onto the freeway headed in the wrong direction toward your car. The best you can hope for in this situation is that your automatic stress response will help you avoid a crash. On the other hand, you do control the non–life-threatening events that are most typical in everyday life. You don't have to get upset at a traffic light, when someone is rude to you, or because your to-do list is a mile long. Granted, worry is good if it alerts you to trouble and you solve the problem. But if you get stuck in the worry phase, you trick yourself into thinking you're taking action when all you're really doing is stewing in the stress juices. In most cases, you need to seek solutions, not dwell on problems.

2. Set priorities.

If your stress comes from a cluttered life, it's time to simplify. Sit down with paper and pencil and list your priorities. What is most important to you? What adds the most quality to your life? It might be family, home, health, work, or maybe a favorite pet. Your life priorities should be where you spend your time and, hopefully, should be joyful play time. Give up responsibilities that are stealing precious time away from the important things in your life. Don't spend time with people you don't like. Don't frequent restaurants where the waiter is rude. Maximize your spare time by limiting television viewing to five hours a week instead of five hours a day, or by checking your e-mail once a day, instead of every hour. Spend that extra time helping the kids with their homework, exercising, or spending a romantic evening with a loved one. Get rid of the physical clutter, too. Throw out the boxes of junk in the attic or garage. If you buy something new, get rid of something old.

3. If it's not urgent AND important, skip it.

Every time you feel your heart or mind begin to race, ask yourself, "How important and urgent is this, and will it be important in six months?" If so, get busy solving the problem. If not, stop expending valuable energy on things that are not that big a deal. Do daily mental reality checks. For example, remind yourself that no one is getting everything done, on time, and perfectly, so why should you be different? Throw out the all-or-nothing thinking (you're not a failure at parenting just because you yelled at the kids today). When you step back and take an objective look at your thoughts, it may be easy to see how beliefs that the house should always be spotless, you should be ultra-thin or fit, or that a person who works hard should always be successful can add unnecessary pressure to your life.

4. Avoid it or deal with it.

Those are your options when it comes to any problem in life. If you hate doing taxes, avoid them by hiring an accountant. If you tense up in rush-hour traffic, avoid it by arriving and leaving work a half hour earlier. Dealing with a stress can mean changing your job if you hate it, or your attitude about it. You can switch roommates or decide not to react if you don't get along. Avoiding stress also means preventing it from happening. For example, think before you say "yes" to requests.

5. Practice time trust.

Much of our modern-day stress is time-related. We feel like we're in a hurry, even when we're not. If your mantra is "I don't have enough time," then it's likely to be a self-fulfilling prophecy. Instead, create a new mantra, such as "I have abundant time and everything is unfolding perfectly." You'll be surprised how life begins to fall into place. Even if you don't get everything done, you won't be so harried in the process. Simplifying your life and trusting that you have enough time also helps you slow down and enjoy life more.

6. Take care of yourself.

People who eat and exercise in tune with their evolutionary heritage cope better with stress. As mentioned in chapter 6, exercise is the natural way to effectively burn off stress hormones and return the body to a calm state. One person who adopted the Origin Diet and Workout Program said it well: "I can be fretting about something that seems so important, but after I've had a great workout, it just doesn't seem that big a deal anymore!"

7. Relax and laugh more.

The relaxation response produces the opposite effect on the body of the stress response, but it doesn't kick in automatically. You must nurture it by planning relaxing moments into your daily schedule. Spending time in nature and with family and friends can evoke the sense of peace associated with relaxation. Laughter suppresses the release of the stress hormones, relaxes muscles, improves breathing and circulation, and oxygenates the blood. Meditation, relaxation exercises, yoga, and deep breathing also help the body unwind. These techniques are most effective if used for prevention, not as treatments. Relaxation techniques aren't the total solution, but they are effective add-ons to the more important business of living life at a slower, more human pace that is in tune with your evolutionary roots.

You also might consider how possessions influence your life. Many people have traded less time for more VCRs, computers, fancy cars, and food processors, items that the rest of the world does fine without. Labor-saving devices—from washing machines and vacuum cleaners to fax machines and hair dryers—were supposed to free more time for leisure, but have only increased our expectations of how much can get done and how clean things should be. If your possessions are running your life, you might consider scaling down your lifestyle. Find ways to live a less affluent life with more time to spend on your priorities. It might mean big changes, like trading in your full-time job for job sharing, switching from a two- to a one-career family, or not buying on credit. It might mean only minor adjustments, such as driving an older car or buying fewer toys, clothes, or appliances. You might be surprised to find you don't need much of what you thought was essential.

Your life is a one-way ticket. Every moment that passes is precious, if only because it will never come again. As you read this paragraph, a minute is slipping through your fingers. If you ignore or rush through the moment, you'll miss your life. Stress numbs you to living and cuts short our few precious years. Reclaim your health, rekindle a passion for living, and breathe joy for the mundane into your life by using the stress response to your favor, not as a lifestyle.

Stone Age Secret #4: Lazy Days Around the Cave and the Importance of Rest, Relaxation, and Quiet Time

The hunting party described above had walked and run for days and had carried both the kill and their wounded for miles over rough terrain back to camp. Now it was time to rest. Even modern-day hunter-gatherers spend only about nineteen hours a week in vigorous activity. Much of the remaining time is spent visiting with loved ones, resting, relaxing, and working on necessary and artistic projects. It's no wonder that our bodies today also need rest and relaxation, time to ponder, create, sleep, and enjoy the company of close friends.

Rest is a vital part of the Stone Age Secrets. It kept our ancient ancestors alert and gave them a competitive edge on survival. Relaxation is one of the Original Dozen, because it provides balance to vigorous activity. Throughout history, those who took time to rest and sleep felt better, thought faster, stayed healthier, and lived longer than their overworked, sleep-deprived camp mates. They also handled stress more effectively, so were more prepared to survive an attack by a lioness, out-smart an enemy, woo a good mate, raise more children, and live into old age to pass on their knowledge to the next generation. Rest provides the same benefits to us today. As with our ancient ancestors, we are more productive and happier when we're rested.

SLEEPLESS ON THE SAVANNA

Sleep deprivation is not the fabric of survival. Sleep loss is the culprit in many car accidents, train and air crashes, nuclear disasters, and industrial catastrophes. "Sleep deprivation has effects on the body much like stress, including weight gain, increased cortisol levels, distorted thyroid hormone levels, and elevations in glucose and insulin that increase the risk for insulin resistance and diabetes," says Robert Sack, Ph.D., at the Oregon Health Sciences University in Portland. Groggy people are short on memory, poor decision makers, low on motivation, and they handle stress poorly. They stumble with vocabulary and communication, are accident prone, and have trouble learning, reasoning, analyzing, or calculating. Failure to get enough sleep also makes them drowsy, fatigued, depressed, irritable, stressed, and antisocial. Being tired undermines relationships and has even ruined marriages. It is also related to weight gain, since tired people often turn to food as an aid for staying awake. A study from the University of Pennsylvania School of Medicine in Philadelphia found that when people's sleep was limited to five hours a night for seven nights, they first felt fatigued and showed reduced reaction times on mental tests. By the third day, they had trouble staying awake or concentrating, their joints were sore, and they experienced headaches, digestive tract problems, irritability, and depression. The researchers concluded that the harmful effects of sleep deprivation are cumulative.

Sleep deprivation suppresses our immune systems, so we're more prone to colds, infections, and disease. Just one bad night can reduce the activity of immune cells called natural killer (NK) cells, according to a study from the San Diego Veterans Affairs Medical Center. The healthy adults in this study were allowed to sleep peacefully for two nights, but on the third night they were awakened at 3:00 A.M. and were kept awake until the next night. As a result, NK cell activity dropped 30 percent, leaving people vulnerable to infections the following day and potentially prolonging recovery from illness, surgery, and colds. Chronic sleep deprivation has even more dramatic effects, including hallucinations, delusions, slowed reflexes, poor judgment, and feelings of paranoia and hostility.

With so much at stake, it's no wonder that half the world's people nap between one and four every afternoon! This inclination to snooze probably dates back to the days on the hot savanna, where our ancestors learned to concentrate their activity in the cooler morning and evening hours, while resting during the hottest time of the day. People who nap have overall better moods than non-nappers, reflecting our inherent need to take a midday break.

EVEN EDUCATED FLEAS DO IT

All animals rest. "We don't have all the answers as to why sleep has such as restorative effect on the body and mind," says Dr. Sack. What we do know is:

- Most growth, repair, recuperation, and recovery occurs during sleep, especially deep sleep, where the body restores organs, bones, and tissues and boosts levels of circulating growth hormone, a hormone essential in muscle repair. Granted, the body repairs muscle throughout the day, but without the extra dose of growth hormone stimulated during deep sleep, less muscle is built. For example, weight lifters lose significant amounts of strength after only two restless nights.
- The immune system kicks into high gear during sleep to kill off bacteria and other disease-causing germs.
- It's during sleep that our bodies generate adenosine triphosphate (ATP), the quick-energy currency of the body that allows us to think and move fast. When people don't sleep well, adenosine accumulates in the tissues, contributing to loss of mental and physical function.

It's no surprise that depriving your body of rest means suppressing its natural ability to repair and defend itself.

Sleep quality is even more important than quantity. About one quarter of a night is spent in rapid eye movement (REM) sleep, which is a light sleep phase where your eyes dart around, the heart rate fluctuates, and dreaming occurs. The other 75 percent is non-REM, much of which is a deep sleep where the body sinks into a hibernation-like state. REM serves an important role in learning, problem solving, and how we process information. Non-REM is the time when our batteries are recharged and our physical energy is restored. We don't feel rested when we miss getting enough non-REM or when the balance between the two phases is disrupted.

HOW DO YOU KNOW IF YOU'RE RESTED?

Our bodies thrive on rest, relaxation, and sleep. Yet, more than half of us are sleep deprived. Most don't even know they need more shuteye. People who brag that they only need five or six hours of sleep a night actually sleep eight or more hours like everyone else when placed in isolation without clocks. Many of us harbor years of accumulated sleep debt and don't even know it. We've grown accustomed to marginal alertness, assuming it's normal to feel this way, when actually we're functioning well below our maximum alertness where we optimize our creativity, happiness, productivity, health, and enthusiasm.

Our modern-day lifestyles interfere with rest. From following fad diets, vitamin or mineral deficiencies, and drinking coffee to stress, smoking, obesity, and overexercise, we make choices that undermine a good night's sleep. We also work too much. In the past twenty years, Americans have added 158 more hours to their annual work and commute schedules, the equivalent of a month's worth of 40-hour work weeks! The time must come from somewhere, and, in many cases, it comes from our sleep and rest time. In the past one hundred years, our average total sleep has dwindled 2 percent. Although Americans spend mindless hours in front of the television, less time is spent in leisure activities that restore our passion for living, whether it's laughing with friends, playing an instrument, taking a walk in the woods, or reading a novel.

Other aspects of our modern-day lives also interfere with restful activity and sound sleep. Working women who shoulder more than their share of household duties forfeit precious relaxation time by working the equivalent of two full-time jobs. Noise pollution—from traffic and trains to airplanes, machinery, loud music, and city life—is in stark contrast to the silence of nature and can interfere with relaxation. Start looking at your world in terms of what enhances your peace of mind and what disrupts it. Then develop a plan for refining your environment and life to nurture relaxation.

Take, for example, our well-lit lives. Artificial lighting in the evening could upset some people's natural sleep/wake cycles, shifting their internal clocks and producing sleep problems much like jet lag. Compared to our Paleolithic ancestors, who rose at sunrise and went to bed at sunset, we rise before dawn by alarm clocks, schedule our lives around deadlines, and turn on the lights and TV when it's dark outside. In a study from Harvard, people were exposed to different levels of light to see if it affected their body temperatures, an indicator of where people are in their circadian cycles. Normally, body temperature drops in the evening and rises in the morning. But in this study, even normal room light shifted the people's body temperatures and their circadian rhythms. The brighter the light and the longer the people sat by lights, the bigger the shift in body rhythm, much the same as what happens when we are outdoors in the sunshine. Not everyone is affected, but if you have trouble sleeping or typically wake up tired, you might be sensitive to the effects of artificial lights.

RESTFUL NIGHTS

How do you know if you need more sleep? If you think you're a good sleeper because you fall asleep as soon as your head hits the pillow, think again. This is the first sign of sleep deprivation. Well-rested people take fifteen to twenty minutes to fall asleep. You also might be sleep deprived if you are drowsy when driving or fall asleep in front of the TV, while relaxing after dinner, during meetings, or in a warm room. On the other hand, if you wake before the alarm goes off and feel rested, then you're probably getting enough sleep. If you find little or no time to read, sit quietly, pursue a creative hobby, visit with friends, or nap, you are rest-deprived, regardless of how much sleep you get.

Ideally, we should go to bed when we're tired and rise every morning when we're fully rested and without the aid of alarm clocks. For those who can't live this vacation lifestyle, here are a few sleep boosters to help you get the rest you need:

- Sleep late on weekends and on days off.
- Take a twenty-minute catnap in the early afternoon before 3:00 P.M. Later naps make it difficult to sleep well at night.
- If you can't nap, take ten-minute "time-outs" from work or daily routine to relax and refresh your mind.
- Exercise in the morning. Vigorous activity within three hours of bedtime can disrupt sleep.
- Watch out for caffeine and other stimulants and avoid alcohol. Even a cup of coffee midafternoon could keep you up at night. Alcohol disrupts quality sleep, so you don't feel rested in the morning.
- Don't smoke. Nicotine is a stimulant.
- Make sure you sleep on a comfortable mattress.
- Use white-noise makers or earplugs if you live in a noisy neighborhood or with a snoring spouse. They produce soothing sounds to mask other noises. Some have natural sounds that mimic the ocean, rivers, waterfalls, rain, or birds chirping.
- Practice relaxation techniques, such as meditation or deep breathing.
- Eat a light evening meal. Heavy meals make you groggy and interfere with deep sleep.
- Eat an all-carbohydrate snack an hour before bedtime, such as a toasted whole grain English muffin with honey, air-popped popcorn, half a whole wheat bagel with jam, or two whole wheat fig bars. Carbohydrates raise brain levels of a nerve chemical called serotonin, which helps you sleep.
- Establish relaxing pre-sleep rituals, such as taking a hot bath before bed to relax tense muscles and raise body temperature. Go to bed at the same time every night.

- If you haven't fallen asleep after thirty minutes, get up and read or listen to soft music in a darkened room. Go to bed when you feel sleepy.

Fresh Air: Build an Environment Suited to Your Ancient Roots

Take a moment and close your eyes. Take a few deep breaths, then visualize a calm scene, one where you feel at peace, refreshed, and fully alive.

You probably had visions of sitting by the ocean, in the wilderness or forest, at the top of a high mountain overlooking the world, lying in the grass staring up at a starry sky, or some other natural scene. Seldom does anyone visualize themselves in rush-hour traffic, waiting in a long line, or sitting at a desk in a windowless office.

Our origins are in nature. We evolved from and in it. It is our home. It soothes us and restores the natural rhythm to our lives. We return to our true natures, are at home in our skin, and are innately soothed by the open range. "Nature shifts our bodies into a more harmonious rhythm; it slows us down and moves us deeper into ourselves," says Faye Snider, M.S.W., and a founding member of the Ecopsychology Institute, the Center for Psychology and Social Change in Cambridge, Massachusetts. The sight of majestic trees, flowing streams, rugged mountains, endless valleys, or the colors at sunrise awaken our senses. The smell of fresh-cut grass, a meadow in springtime, or sea air eases our minds. The sound of rain, ocean waves crashing on the shore, or wind whistling through branches arouses our spirits just as they must have aroused the spirits of our ancient ancestors.

People who spend time in the fresh air and sunshine sleep better at night and are more successful at handling stress. Blood cholesterol levels drop in the summer when people work outdoors in their gardens, then rise in the winter when they shut themselves indoors. A variety of emotional, mental, and anxiety disorders improve when people spend time outdoors. Hospital patients whose windows look out on trees and plants recover quicker and need fewer medications for pain than do patients who view brick walls. Most people also enjoy nature programs on television.

Richard Coss, Ph.D., at the University of California, Davis, studied the effects of nature scenes on patients awaiting surgery. "We placed calming, serene scenes of mountains, water, and open spaces above the lighting units so that patients could view them just before entering surgery. Blood pressures dropped as a result," says Dr. Coss. Interestingly, patients who viewed pictures of sailboarding, paddling, or wild animals experienced elevated blood pressures. "Even though these pictures were beautiful and the animals were not threatening, these pictures aroused the patients, rather than calming them," says Dr. Coss.

Why does nature soothe us? Dr. Coss suspects that as long as there are no immediate dangers, such as a grizzly bear or snakes, then natural landscapes that include water and trees evoke a sense of safety and refuge. "We have an innate attraction to water, and glistening surfaces are especially appealing because they promise that water is readily available. People also are attracted to landscapes with trees because the foliage provides shade and places to hide from predation," continues Dr. Coss. The need for safety, according to the renowned psychologist Abraham Maslow, is one of our most basic and primitive drives. It's no wonder, then, that the security we feel when looking out over a valley with creeks and clusters of trees, when walking in the California redwood forest, or while sitting on a cliff overlooking the ocean soothes us deep down to our evolutionary core.

UNNATURAL LIVING

We have a spiritual and physical dependence on the great outdoors. Theodore Roszak, in his book *The Voice of the Earth* (Simon and Schuster, 1992), states that while we give much attention to separation anxiety disorders as they pertain to the excessive stress concerning separation from home and from those we love, we often fail to realize that no separation is as profound as a disconnection from nature.

"We are caught up in an unnatural rhythm today, one dominated by machines. When we leave that hectic pace and spend time in a natural setting, even if it's only to meander in a garden or walk a local trail, we resonate to a life pulse that is familiar and natural to our bodies," says

Snider. If we live without fresh air and natural surroundings, our spirits wither. Air pollution in big cities alone aggravates bronchitis, asthma, and other lung disorders in children and adults, increases the need for hospital and physician services and medications, is responsible for lost wages, and increases mortality rates, especially for lung cancer and heart disease. Imagine the total cost that living apart from nature must have on our spirits, lives, and health!

Our ancestors lived their lives outdoors; today we spend up to 95 percent of our time indoors. They had grass and dirt beneath their feet; we have rubber soles, carpet, and concrete. They felt the breeze on their faces and smelled the changes of seasons; we live cushioned from our senses by one-inch insulated windowpanes and temperature-controlled buildings. "People are naturally attracted to the growth, beauty, and serenity they find in nature. We thrive in that outdoors. Our senses attune to the quieter rhythms. Our bodies and minds calm down. You see it on the faces of families when they're at the beach or when hiking. They're more relaxed and open," says Snider.

When we trade time in nature for more time indoors, we also expose ourselves to indoor pollutants for which we have no natural defense. In one study, levels of air pollutants in the home were five to seventy times higher than the highest outdoor levels. The consequences to our health include flulike symptoms, headaches, fatigue, irritated eyes, coughing, skin rashes, aggravated asthma and chronic diseases, chemical-sensitivity syndrome, and dizziness. Office buildings can be just as hazardous, with air pollution levels accumulating to levels high enough to cause sick building syndrome, characterized by headaches, poor concentration, chest tightness, shortness of breath, reduced work performance, and fatigue.

Besides animal dander, dust, fibrous glass particles, mold spores, germs, and mites, common pollutants in our homes and workplaces include:

- benzene from attached garages,
- carbon monoxide from fireplaces and heaters,
- chloroform from washing machines,

- formaldehyde from pressed wood products and permanent-press draperies,
- polyaromatic hydrocarbons (PAHs) from candles and charbroiling meats,
- paradichlorobenzene from air fresheners, mothballs, and bathroom deodorizers,
- perchloroethylene from freshly dry-cleaned clothes,
- pesticides from flea powders, pet shampoos, and garden pesticides tracked in on shoes, and
- radon, a radioactive element that seeps from the earth and is known to cause lung cancer.

Well-insulated, energy-efficient homes where windows and doors are kept shut are the most likely candidates for high indoor air pollution.

A BREATH OF FRESH AIR

We should heed the cues from our ancient ancestors and take nature more seriously. Your emotional, mental, and physical health depends on it in the short run, and the survival of our species, if not the entire planet, depends on it long-term.

- Include some outdoor activity in your daily schedule, even if it's only to walk to the mailbox or roll down the windows of your car.
- At least once a week, plan an outdoor activity, such as bike riding, a walk or hike in the country or the park, a game of basketball with the kids, ice skating or swimming, a stroll on the beach, or a canoe ride.
- Put away the Walkman, the watch, and the pedometer and take a no-distractions walk.
- When outside, awaken your senses by paying attention to smells, sights, colors, sounds, and the feel of the sun or snowflakes on your skin. Listen to the wind, the birds, and the leaves crackling underfoot. Smell the wet leaves in the fall, the snow in the winter, the fragrances after a spring rain, and the warm air in summer. You'll find that many of the day's stresses melt away when your senses are piqued by the outdoors.

- Bring the outdoors into your daily life with windows that open onto the garden, fountains, wind chimes, sun roofs or solar tubes, plants, and fragrances, such as pine, apple, roses, and citrus. Use dimmer switches and candles.

- Protect nature. Avoid pesticides in your garden. Buy organic food when possible. Invest in environmentally protective companies. Support or join groups who are protecting the environment.

- If you live in a large city, exercise in the morning when air pollution levels are low. Keep kids indoors on smoggy days.

- Keep your home and workspace well ventilated by opening windows whenever possible. Even in cold weather, you can open a window a crack. Use fans that vent to the outdoors, especially in the kitchen, bathrooms, and any room with a fireplace or wood stove. Open doors between rooms. See the box below for other ideas on how to keep your home free from pollutants.

HOME, CLEAN HOME

"There's no place like home," said Dorothy in *The Wizard of Oz.* That's true only if your home is the safe haven it should be, not one riddled with pollutants. Here's a list of ideas for minimizing the health hazards in your home:

- Don't smoke and don't allow smoking in your home or office.
- In the kitchen, use the stove fan or open a window. Cooking is the second leading cause of indoor air pollution.
- Skip the air fresheners. They contain organic chemicals that quickly vaporize and might cause cancer.
- Use scented candles and potpourris only when windows are open.
- Don't use mothballs. Instead, clean clothing before storing, dry-clean woolens and linens. Store clothing and fabrics in airtight containers.
- Air dry-cleaned clothes outdoors if they smell of chemicals.

- Wash permanent-press clothes and fabrics before using.
- Use a good doormat that will remove as much dirt and pollutants as possible from your shoes.
- Vacuum floors and rugs frequently.
- Install low-emissions carpeting and padding in your home.
- Avoid hair sprays, nail polish, and spray perfumes or use only in vented areas.
- Keep your home free of lead by using lead-free paint, hiring a contractor to remove existing lead-based paint, and having your drinking water tested for lead.
- Frequently clean your air conditioner filter.
- Ventilate your attic to prevent moisture buildup.
- Replace moldy shower curtains in the bathroom.
- Empty and clean refrigerator condensation trays.
- Clean and dry water-damaged rugs and carpets immediately to prevent mold and mildew.
- Test for radon. If levels are too high, hire a certified radon contractor to fix the problem, by sealing cracks in a basement, for example.

Stone Age Secret #5: Belong to a Supportive Tribe of Family and Friends

Imagine that you are part of the welcoming party 40,000 years ago that greeted the returning hunters described above. You were born into a nomadic tribe of 50 to 150 people. You've known everyone in the clan intimately your entire life. As a baby, you never went without physical contact, being strapped to your mother during the day and sleeping with family members at night. As an adult, you know how everyone is related to you. Some you love deeply, and you're loved deeply in return. Others you are not especially fond of, but you know them well enough to know what to expect. You also know exactly what everyone expects from you. Life in the wild might be unpredictable, but within your social world, the rules are clear, crime is minimal (it's impossible to get away with anything when everyone knows you!), and you feel a strong sense of belonging, which lets you feel safe and secure.

Our evolutionary success depended on more than big brains, opposable thumbs, and upright posture. In a harsh and dangerous world, our species survived and evolved because of our amazing social skills at relying, supporting, cooperating, and knowing whom to trust and whom to watch closely. It doesn't take an Einstein to find food and shelter; all animals do that. Our ancestors banded together to do what no individual could have done alone and no other species has done before or since, from coordinating hunting parties and surviving ice ages to developing tools, painting masterpieces, and creating complex social and political systems. Alone, an ancient ancestor would have starved or become prey. Together *Homo sapiens* took over the world. Each of us harbors that ancient social legacy. Our basic need for security, safety, and love is met, in part, by belonging to a supportive group.

Our brains are the product of millions of years of evolution that customized us to cooperate with small, well-known bands of people. Our ancient ancestors rarely knew more than about 150 people, which interestingly is the maximum most people have in their immediate circles today. The complexities of forging relationships with the thousands of people who come into our lives on the street, the television, or the Internet is more than our Paleolithic minds can handle. No wonder impersonal bureaucracies, voice messaging systems, rudeness from strangers, and telemarketers are so maddening. How alien to the world in which we evolved!

SOCIAL OUTCASTS

Do you know anyone (including yourself) who has lived in the same neighborhood and known the same neighbors for generations? Whom do you know who has kept the same job and has gone regularly to the same church or synagogue for decades? Do you know anyone who has lived within a mile of extended family their entire lives? Who, when raising children with the help of extended family, never owned a crib or stroller, but instead kept their babies physically close until they could walk? Do you have even one friend who is well known by almost everyone he or she passes on the street?

In stark contrast to our evolutionary roots, we live hundreds of miles from family, move from city to city and job to job, leave friends behind, and are bombarded with nonstop information about strangers. We are surrounded by more people we don't know than ever before in the history of humankind. Yet without the small band of lifelong friends, many people live their lives unheard and unseen. Many have nowhere to feel special, known, and understood. Without loving relationships, many people today lack intimacy. They feel isolated and alone, which brings with it a host of physical, emotional, and spiritual ills. "A lack of social support is a type of stress; both share many of the same consequences, such as illness and depression," says James Pennebaker, Ph.D., at the University of Texas in Austin.

We derive an inner peace when we're with friends and family who are truly interested in us, who know our faults, yet love and admire us anyway. "Friends and loving family members give us a place to seek help, someone to talk to, somewhere to vent, all of which has a positive effect on our physical health," says Dr. Pennebaker.

LOVE AND HEALTH

We are social creatures, so it's not surprising that anything that connects us with others in caring relationships helps us navigate through life, reduces stress, and keeps us grounded. "In the past twenty years, there have been hundreds of studies showing that the stronger people's social support, the better their health," says Dr. Pennebaker. Any choice we make that promotes isolation contributes to illness and poor quality of life. Any choice that promotes feelings of belonging, connectedness, and community is innately satisfying and healing. Caring produces emotional, physical, and spiritual results.

Depression ranks fourth among health problems worldwide and is projected to rise to second place by 2020. Depression rates are rising especially fast in young adults. A major factor in this epidemic is believed to be the demise of family and social connectedness. A number of studies show that people who maintain strong social ties cope better with stress (such as bereavement, job loss, and illness) and are much less likely to battle depression, suicide, drug abuse, and alcoholism than people who feel socially isolated. Strong, loving relationships formed early in life allow children to grow up self-confident and able to cope. Teenagers in supportive, communicative families are happier, less stressed, and more confident than teenagers who feel alone. Adults, especially women, in loving marriages and with close confidants have low rates of depression and illness. In contrast, a lack of supportive friends and family contributes to depression. "In our research on HIV-infected men, we found that men with high levels of social conflict and little social support in their lives were most prone to mood disorders and depression," says Jane Leserman, Ph.D., research associate professor at the University of North Carolina.

Caring has physical effects. People who feel isolated and lonely have three to five times the rates of premature death and age-related disease as people who feel loved and connected to other people. Nurturing relationships also improve overall health, boost immunity, speed recovery from surgery and illness, help us live long lives, and even boost our weight-loss efforts. Those people who help others, in turn, live longer.

Dr. Leserman found that men infected with HIV who had the most support from friends and family had the lowest rates of progression to AIDS. "The benefits of social support were cumulative, with disease risk dropping as support increased," says Dr. Leserman. Disease and death rates from all causes also are lowest in towns where people have strong ties to family, traditions, or culture. As those ties loosen, the community spirit weakens and death rates increase, especially for heart disease.

There appears to be a connection between stress and isolation, since both stress and lack of support escalate disease progression. A lack of social connectedness raises levels of stress hormones, such as cortisol, which further damages tissues. In studies on rats, isolated animals exposed to stresses are more likely to die than are animals exposed to the same stress but who live with littermates. However, the mechanism by which isolation leads to disease in people is poorly understood, since the connection between cortisol and isolation has not been verified.

WOMEN ARE GATHERERS,
MEN ARE HUNTERS

My father had a gun case with a glass door. When my daughter and son were little, they would independently stop in front of that gun case. My daughter used the glass as a mirror to primp. My son gazed covetously at the guns inside. Same gun case, two totally different experiences.

Women and men are more alike than not, but the few distinctions are very noticeable and find their origins in our ancient histories. Many anthropologists speculate that, as gatherers, women evolved skills to find the best stationary foods. They learned to remember details of the environment: by what tree the best berries were found, where the largest roots were buried, and when they would be ready to dig, or by what rock downstream were the crawdads. In contrast, men hunted moving game. They evolved linear thinking and learned to navigate by creating a mental map of the overall pattern of their world.

Today, women remain diffuse thinkers, using more compartments of their brains to problem-solve than men. As a result, they far outperform men in remembering details of their environment, from objects in a room to landmarks on a road trip. "Women give you directions based on landmarks. They tell you to turn at the blue house or just past the lilac tree. On the other hand, men describe their location in terms of direction and distance, so they're more apt to tell you to drive two blocks then turn north," says Dr. Richard Coss. Maybe that's why men won't ask for directions if lost, since they rely on a sense of movement, not landmarks, to judge their course.

Women evolved more precise skills for interpreting nonverbal communication. Both men and women are adept at reading happy faces, but women far out outperform men when it comes to sad emotions. Men miss the subtleties and only recognize sadness on a woman's face if that expression is extreme. Women's brains are slightly smaller, but the areas of higher thinking, especially language, are more densely packed with nerve cells. The connecting tissue that links the right (the emotional/intuitive) and left (rational/logical) hemispheres of the brain is thicker in women than in men. In contrast, men's brains respond in highly specialized areas to think through problems.

The differences go on and on. Neither style of thinking is better or worse, just different, reflecting the skills needed to find food, raise children, and survive in a harsh world. So next time your partner is driving you crazy, remember, what he or she is doing or saying might have saved your life 40,000 years ago!

People who combine strong social support with spiritual beliefs by regularly attending church or synagogue have one fourth the risk of developing hypertension, a 50 percent lower risk for developing heart disease, and significantly less overall illness, and they have 28 percent lower risk of dying prematurely as people who do not attend church. The more people feel connected and loved, the healthier they are. For example:

• In a study from the University of Texas Medical School, patients waiting for open-heart surgery were asked if they were members of social groups who met regularly (bowling league, bingo group, etc.) and if they gained spiritual strength from their religious faith. Those who answered "no" to both questions were seven times more likely to die within six months of surgery compared to those who answered "yes."

• A study from Duke University found that adults who were not married and who didn't have close friends to share thoughts, worries, and ideas were three times more likely than their more socially connected friends to die from heart disease.

• Women with breast cancer live the longest when they are regular members of support or religious groups.

• People with few quality social contacts have higher blood pressure, according to a study from the University of Utah.

GET SOCIAL

No other species on earth is as social as people. We grieve for our dead. Lend a hand to strangers. Bond with lovers. Make bosom buddies and cherish kindred spirits. Love to debate, argue, discuss, and share. Friendship is so inherent in our nature that we even talk to God, holler at our cars, tell secrets to our pets, and scold the weather. The intimacy, belonging, connectedness, and admiration that come from loving relationships are as essential to our self-worth and survival as is the air we breathe. As Dr. Leserman says, "We need to be touched just as we need food." We must give and receive love to feel truly human.

The dining table is a wonderful way to nourish our social natures. Throughout our history, food has provided joyous opportunities to connect with one another, spend time with family and loved ones, and to feel secure, safe, and loved. Turn off the TV at mealtime. Rekindle family traditions, such as birthday parties, holiday get-togethers, and family dinners. Nurture the connection with past generations by serving family recipes. Start new family traditions. These rituals link us to our families and our past, give us a sense of belonging, and reinforce who we are.

Friends are the pulse of life. They nourish our spirits, our moods, and our health. "Ideally, long-term friendships are the best, but even new friendships improve our health if those friendships are based on trust," says Dr. Pennebaker. Dr. Leserman agrees, adding that it's not so much the number of friends a person has, but the quality of those friendships that seems to cushion us from disease.

The bottom line is to nurture quality friendships, regardless of whether they are lifelong or short-lived. Let down your guard so friendships can grow beyond the superficial. Share worries and joys, ask for advice, and help others. How you communicate will either push people away or bring them closer. Accept people, don't criticize them. Be assertive in your communication, not passive or aggressive. Be honest, direct, and loving in your communication. Listen carefully to others. Acknowledge and express feelings. Forgive and forget. Touch those you love by hugging more, giving more shoulder rubs, and holding their hands.

Expand your social horizons. If you already have a few best buddies, add more people to your inner world by reaching out to neighbors, club members, and workmates. If you're new to an area, join a church or social group. If you already belong to a group, increase your participation. Join a reading group. Stay in touch with family. Help others through volunteer work. Baby-sit for someone who is housebound. Shovel a neighbor's sidewalk. Put a dime in a stranger's parking meter. Buy someone flowers. Read more to children (storytelling is especially soothing, probably because it has been a part of our heritage since the development of language). What's important is that your social connections give you a haven where you can communicate, vent, be heard and helped, offer help to others, explore thoughts, and feel understood.

A Truly Human Life

The cardiologist and runner Dr. George Sheehan once said, "Heed the inner calling to your own play . . . something that gives you security and self-acceptance and a feeling of completion. . . . When you find it, build your life around it." We must strive to nurture lives that are in balance with and that fulfill the needs of our ancient biology. It is when we honor that heritage by embracing pastimes that bring us innate peace of mind and a feeling of connectedness to our community and families today and to future generations that we truly soothe our souls, heal our bodies and minds, and invigorate our relationships.

Appendix

A Five-Day Meal Plan, plus Menus for Breakfast, Lunch, and Dinner

The Original Five-Day Meal Plan

Eating in tune with your evolutionary roots is easy, just include lots of fruits and vegetables at every meal and snack, load up on other phytochemical-rich goodies, like fresh herbs, garlic, nuts, and soy, then lace the menu with very lean meat, such as fish, shellfish, or the white meat of poultry. Drink lots of water, sweeten with dried fruits and honey, and—of course—exercise daily! (Even though the following menus are loaded with vitamins and minerals, you still might consider taking a moderate-dose multiple vitamin and mineral supplement, plus extra vitamin E and fish oils.) Recipes for the dishes with asterisks can be found starting on page 247.

DAY 1

BREAKFAST

⅔ cup oatmeal cooked in 1 cup vanilla-flavored soymilk and topped with

> *2 tablespoons toasted wheat germ*
>
> *2 tablespoons raisins*
>
> *2 tablespoons chopped walnuts*

1 cup orange juice
1 banana
Herb or green tea

MIDMORNING SNACK

1 cup nonfat plain yogurt mixed with

> *2 tablespoons chopped dates*
> *1 tablespoon chopped almonds*

Iced green tea or water

LUNCH

Thai Tofu Salad (serve hot or cold):

3 ounces firm tofu, cut into cubes and heated in a nonstick pan for 5 minutes. Add 2 cups preshredded cabbage mix, 1 tablespoon peanut sauce, and 1 tablespoon sunflower seeds. Heat over medium heat for 2 minutes (or until heated through, but still crunchy). Top with ¼ cup chopped fresh cilantro and serve.

2 medium tomatoes, sliced and topped with

> *2 minced garlic cloves*
> *2 tablespoons chopped fresh basil*
> *1 teaspoon balsamic vinegar*

Sparkling water with lemon or herb tea

MIDAFTERNOON SNACK

1 cup nonfat milk blended with

> *1 teaspoon nutmeg*
> *1 teaspoon honey*
> *1 ice cube*

DINNER

4 ounces roast chicken breast (stuff chicken with fresh rosemary and onions before roasting)

Glazed Carrots:

2 carrots, peeled and sliced into ¼-inch diagonals, cooked in 1 teaspoon olive oil and ⅓ cup orange juice until tender. In a small bowl, mix until smooth ½ teaspoon cornstarch, ¼ teaspoon ground ginger, pinch of nutmeg, and 3 tablespoons water. Add ginger mixture to carrots and stir over medium heat until sauce thickens. Sprinkle with 2 teaspoons chopped chives and a pinch of red pepper flakes (optional).

1 cup steamed Brussels sprouts
1 cup mashed parsnips topped with ¼ teaspoon ground nutmeg
Sparkling water with lime juice

EVENING SNACK

2 cups frozen grapes
Water

Nutritional information: 1,943 calories, 23 percent fat (51 grams), 57 percent carbohydrate, 20 percent protein, 44 grams fiber, 1,301 milligrams calcium

DAY 2

BREAKFAST

Veggie Omelet:

Whip 1 whole egg and 2 egg whites and pour into nonstick 10-inch frying pan coated with vegetable spray. Cover and cook over medium heat until cooked through and firm. Remove in one piece, place on plate, fill with steamed vegetables (onions, garlic, zucchini, mushrooms, red peppers, etc.) and fresh herbs. Fold egg mixture over vegetable-herb mixture to form an omelet.

1 slice whole wheat bread, toasted, topped with

> *1 tablespoon apricot preserves*

6 ounces grapefruit juice
Herb or green tea

MIDMORNING SNACK

1 cup nonfat milk
1 banana

LUNCH

Black Bean Burrito:

1 whole wheat tortilla, warmed and filled with

> *½ cup black beans, cooked (or canned and drained)*
> *¼ cup brown rice*
> *1 ounce fat-free cheddar cheese, grated*
> *3 tablespoons chopped canned green chilies*
> *3 tablespoons chopped fresh cilantro*
> *2 tablespoons bottled enchilada sauce*

And topped with

> *2 tablespoons fat-free sour cream*
> *3 tablespoons salsa*

1 medium orange, cut into wedges
½ papaya, peeled and cut into slices
Iced tea

MIDAFTERNOON SNACK

⅓ cup hummus

1 carrot, peeled and cut into sticks

⅓ cup jicama, peeled and cut into strips

Water or herb or green tea

DINNER

Ginger Barbecued Salmon,* 1 serving

1 cup wild rice with 2 tablespoons almond slivers

15 mushrooms, sautéed in ¼ cup chicken broth with 3 cloves garlic, minced

Roasted Lemon Asparagus and Red Peppers,* 1 serving

Sparkling water, herb tea, or water

EVENING SNACK

1 cup nonfat milk, warmed and flavored with

almond extract and nutmeg

1 cup blueberries

Nutritional information: 1,965 calories, 21 percent fat (46 grams), 59 percent carbohydrate, 20 percent protein, 55 grams fiber, 967 milligrams calcium

DAY 3

BREAKFAST

1 whole wheat waffle topped with

2 teaspoons fat-free cream cheese

2 teaspoons marmalade (preferably made with honey)

1 tangerine, peeled, sectioned, and seeded

⅓ honeydew melon, drizzled with

lime juice

And topped with

  1 fresh mint sprig

1 cup vanilla-flavored fat-free soymilk

MIDMORNING SNACK

2 plums

1 cup nonfat milk, blended with vanilla, nutmeg, and an ice cube

LUNCH

1 cup Hearty Barley Mushroom Soup*

1 sweet potato, cut into quarters and baked at 350°F until tender on the inside and crunchy on the outside (approximately 35 minutes, or 15 minutes in a microwave). Serve hot or cold.

½ cup coleslaw

Sparkling water or herb or green tea

MIDAFTERNOON SNACK

1 baked apple, stuffed with

  2 tablespoons chopped walnuts

  ½ teaspoon ground cinnamon

  2 teaspoons honey

Iced herb or green tea

DINNER

Herb-Rubbed Chicken,* 1 serving

Spinach with a Zing:

In a medium skillet, add 2 tablespoons chicken broth, 2 teaspoons balsamic vinegar, 1 teaspoon olive oil, 1 tablespoon dried cranberries, 2 minced cloves garlic, and a dash of red pepper flakes and nutmeg.

Bring to a simmer. Add ⅓ pound fresh spinach, washed and stemmed. Toss and cook until spinach is wilted, about 1 to 3 minutes.

Papaya-Carrot Salad:

Top 2 cups leaf lettuce with 1 grated carrot and ½ sliced papaya. Mix 1 tablespoon raspberry vinegar and 1 tablespoon canola oil, then pour over salad. Top with 5 fresh red raspberries and 1 teaspoon lemon zest.

1 cup nonfat milk

EVENING SNACK

Late-night sweet treat:

> *1 banana, sliced*
>
> *3 apricot halves, canned in juice and drained*
>
> *2 teaspoons honey*

Nutritional information: 1,984 calories, 25 percent fat (56 grams), 57 percent carbohydrate, 18 percent protein, 41 grams fiber, 1,155 milligrams calcium

DAY 4

BREAKFAST

The Stone Age Zinger Smoothie,* 1 serving

MIDMORNING SNACK

1 oatmeal–raisin cookie
1 cup nonfat milk

LUNCH

Grilled Tofu and Vegetables over Rice:

Marinate in ½ cup chicken broth, 2 tablespoons soy sauce, 5 minced cloves garlic, and 1 tablespoon grated fresh ginger, then grill or roast the following:

4 ounces firm tofu, cut into cubes

1 red bell pepper, seeded and cut into strips

1 yellow bell pepper, seeded and cut into strips

½ onion, sliced

5 mushrooms, sliced

½ cup zucchini rounds

Serve over ½ cup brown rice

Carrot-Apple-Raisin Salad:

2 carrots, peeled and grated

½ apple, cubed

1 tablespoon raisins

1 tablespoon lemon juice

1 tablespoon low-fat mayonnaise

Sparkling water with lemon or herb or green tea

MIDAFTERNOON SNACK

1 cup nonfat milk

1 pear

DINNER

10 large clams, steamed in chicken broth, 5 minced cloves garlic, fresh tarragon, and ½ diced onion

2 whole wheat rolls (dunk in clam juice)

Tossed Salad:

> *2 cups romaine lettuce, chopped*
>
> *1 medium tomato, sliced*
>
> *¼ cup julienned beets*
>
> *2 tablespoons sprouts*
>
> *Dressing: 1 tablespoon red wine vinegar and 1 tablespoon olive oil*

1 cup sparkling apple juice

EVENING SNACK

1 serving Maple Baked Apples with Toasted Oats and Almonds*
Sparkling water

Nutritional information: 1,954 calories, 18 percent fat (39 grams), 64 percent carbohydrate, 18 percent protein, 37 grams fiber, 1,438 milligrams calcium

DAY 5

BREAKFAST

1 buckwheat pancake topped with

> *1 tablespoon raspberry preserves*
>
> *1 cup fresh red raspberries*

½ cantaloupe with lemon juice and a sprig of fresh mint
1 cup vanilla-flavored low-fat soymilk

MIDMORNING SNACK

1 cup nonfat plain yogurt mixed with

> *2 tablespoons dried fruit*
>
> *2 tablespoons slivered almonds*
>
> *2 tablespoons sunflower seeds*
>
> *1 teaspoon honey*

LUNCH

Turkey Sandwich:

> *4 ounces turkey breast*
> *2 lettuce leaves*
> *2 slices of tomato*
> *1 teaspoon honey mustard*
> *2 slices whole wheat bread*

Tossed Salad:

> *2 cups leaf lettuce, chopped*
> *½ winter pear, sliced*
> *2 tablespoons fat-free vinaigrette dressing*

1 cup tomato juice with a dash of Tabasco sauce

MIDAFTERNOON SNACK

2 large celery stalks filled with

> *1 tablespoon peanut (or almond) butter*

Sparkling water with lemon

DINNER

Prawn Kabobs:

Skewer and barbecue, grill, or broil the following:

> *6 jumbo shrimp, peeled and deveined*
> *2 bell peppers (green, red, orange, or yellow),*
> *cut into strips or 1-inch pieces*
> *½ cup red onions, sliced thick*
> *6 large mushrooms*

½ acorn squash, baked
Sparkling water with lime or herb or green tea

EVENING SNACK

Tropical Fruit Salad:

> *1 papaya, sliced*
>
> *1 cup pineapple chunks*
>
> *3 tablespoons canned mandarin orange slices, drained*
>
> *⅓ cup avocado, sliced*
>
> *1 tablespoon orange zest*
>
> *2 tablespoons low-fat bottled lime salad dressing*

Nutritional information: 1,972 calories, 23 percent fat (51 grams), 57 percent carbohydrate, 20 percent protein, 54 grams fiber, 1,142 milligrams calcium

Menus for Breakfast, Lunch, and Dinner

Mix and match the following breakfasts, lunches, and dinners to make a variety of tasty meal plans.

BREAKFAST IDEAS

BREAKFAST 1

Bagel with Roasted Red Pepper Cream Cheese:

Mash together 2 tablespoons nonfat cream cheese with 1 tablespoon diced (water-packed) roasted red pepper. Spread on small (2-ounce) whole wheat sesame bagel.

1 cup cubed cantaloupe or other melon
8 ounces nonfat milk

Nutritional information: 417 calories, 5 percent fat (2.2 grams), 70 percent carbohydrate, 25 percent protein, 9.8 grams fiber

BREAKFAST 2

Chocolate-Banana-Soy Milkshake:

Combine in a blender 1 cup soymilk, 1 banana, 1 teaspoon each cocoa and honey, 1 teaspoon vanilla extract, and 3 ice cubes (optional). Blend until smooth.

1 whole grain waffle topped with

> *1 tablespoon maple syrup*
>
> *1 teaspoon chopped pecans (or any nut)*

1 cup fresh berries

Herb tea

Nutritional information: 465 calories, 22 percent fat (11.5 grams), 67 percent carbohydrate, 11 percent protein, 10.3 grams fiber

BREAKFAST 3

Potatoes and Egg:

Blanch 2 small, diced red potatoes in rapidly boiling water (about 10 minutes). Drain. Sauté 3 tablespoons diced onion in 1 teaspoon olive oil over medium heat (about 3 minutes). Add potatoes, 1 tablespoon red wine vinegar, a dash of red pepper flakes, and ¼ teaspoon each paprika, salt, and pepper. Cook 2 minutes. Poach one egg in boiling water 3 minutes, until cooked through. Serve over potatoes.

1 slice whole wheat toast with 1 teaspoon all-fruit jam

1 cup orange juice

Nutritional information: 429 calories, 24 percent fat (11.6 grams), 63 percent carbohydrate, 13 percent protein, 5.5 grams fiber

BREAKFAST 4

Broiled Grapefruit:

Top one grapefruit half with 1 teaspoon honey and ¼ teaspoon ground nutmeg. Broil 5 minutes, until golden and bubbly.

Mushrooms and Eggs:

Sauté ⅓ cup diced mushrooms (portobello or shiitake are especially good) in 1 teaspoon olive oil. Add ½ cup egg substitute or 3 egg whites and ¼ teaspoon each dried oregano, salt, and black pepper. Sauté until cooked through (3 to 5 minutes).

½ whole wheat English muffin, toasted and topped with

> *1 tablespoon apple butter or all-fruit jam*

Herb tea

Nutritional information: 317 calories, 26 percent fat (9.1 grams), 51 percent carbohydrate, 23 percent protein, 5.5 grams fiber

BREAKFAST 5

1 whole-grain muffin with raisins and nuts topped with

> *1 tablespoon cashew, almond, soy, or peanut butter*

1 cup pineapple chunks, fresh or canned in own juice
1 kiwi fruit, peeled and sliced
Herb tea

Nutritional information: 477 calories, 34 percent fat (18.3 grams), 56 percent carbohydrate, 10 percent protein, 10.1 grams fiber

BREAKFAST 6

⅔ cup low-fat granola (made with canola oil) topped with

> *2 tablespoons dried fruit bits*
> *2⅓ cups nonfat milk*

½ cantaloupe filled with ½ cup plain, nonfat yogurt and ½ cup berries
Herb tea

Nutritional information: 463 calories, 8 percent fat (4.1 grams), 75 percent carbohydrate, 17 percent protein, 7.5 grams fiber

BREAKFAST 7

Breakfast Burrito:

8-inch whole wheat tortilla filled and heated with

> *½ cup scrambled egg substitute,*
>
> *2 tablespoons salsa*
>
> *3 tablespoons fresh chopped cilantro*

1 cup grapefruit juice

Nutritional information: 281 calories, 15 percent fat (4.8 grams), 59 percent carbohydrate, 26 percent protein, 2.5 grams fiber

BREAKFAST 8

½ whole wheat English muffin, toasted and topped with

> *1 tablespoon nut or soy butter*

1 pear, sliced
1 cup orange juice

Nutritional information: 461 calories, 26 percent fat (13.5 grams), 65 percent carbohydrate, 9 percent protein, 10.0 grams fiber

BREAKFAST 9

The Stone Age Zinger Smoothie*

BREAKFAST 10

Mini Breakfast Pizza:

Slice and toast a whole wheat English muffin. Spread each half with 2 tablespoons of a mixture of low-fat lemon yogurt and fat-free cream cheese. Top with ¼ cup fresh fruit, such as pineapple, mandarin orange slices, fresh strawberries, and/or mango. Sprinkle with nutmeg.

1 cup warmed 1 percent low-fat milk flavored with almond extract and sprinkled with cinnamon. (Whip briefly in blender for added froth.)

Nutritional information: 301 calories, 12 percent fat (3.92 grams), 65 percent carbohydrate, 23 percent protein, 2.3 grams fiber

BREAKFAST 11

Low-Fat Omelet:

Mix 1 whole egg and 1 egg white with ¼ cup fat-free cottage cheese, ¼ teaspoon garlic powder, and salt and pepper to taste. Cook in nonstick pan sprayed with vegetable spray.

1 slice whole wheat bread topped with

> *1 teaspoon all-fruit jam*

1 cup orange juice

Nutritional information: 372 calories, 17 percent fat (7.2 grams), 52 percent carbohydrate, 31 percent protein, 3.35 grams fiber

BREAKFAST 12

Mix 1 cup nonfat plain yogurt with a sliced banana, ½ cup berries, ¼ cup Grape-Nuts, and 1 tablespoon flaxseed meal.

1 cup orange juice

Nutritional information: 497 calories, 5 percent fat (2.62 grams), 78 percent carbohydrate, 17 percent protein, 8.35 grams fiber

BREAKFAST 13

Whole Wheat Pancakes:

Mix 1 teaspoon baking soda into 1½ cups buttermilk in a small bowl and set aside. In a large bowl, combine 1 cup whole wheat flour, 2 teaspoons cinnamon, and 1 tablespoon honey. Add buttermilk mixture, 2 beaten egg whites, and 1½ teaspoons vanilla and blend. Spray a griddle with vegetable spray and ladle pancake mixture onto griddle. (Makes about 8 medium-sized pancakes.) A good topping for these pancakes follows.

Fruit Topping:

Combine 2 cups fresh berries (boysenberries, raspberries, or blueberries) with ⅓ cup apple juice in a small saucepan. Simmer for 5 minutes, then add a blend of 1 tablespoon honey and 1 tablespoon cornstarch. Stir gently until berries thicken. Pour over pancakes.

1 cup orange juice

Nutritional information (per 2 pancakes): 321 calories, 6 percent fat (2.16 grams), 81 percent carbohydrate, 13 percent protein, 6.18 grams fiber

BREAKFAST 14

Top 1 whole wheat bagel cut in half with 2 slices cheddar-style fat-free soy cheese and 2 thick slices of tomato. Microwave for about 30 seconds or until cheese bubbles.

1 cup grapefruit juice

Nutritional information: 345 calories, 14 percent fat (5.47 grams), 68 percent carbohydrate, 18 percent protein, 7.28 grams fiber

BREAKFAST 15

Egg McPita:

Combine ½ cup egg substitute with 2 tablespoons chopped green chilies and salt and pepper to taste. Pour into hot nonstick frying pan coated with vegetable spray. Stir occasionally until set. Spoon eggs into a whole wheat pita cut in half, top with 1 tablespoon salsa and 1 tablespoon chopped cilantro.

½ cantaloupe
1 cup nonfat milk

Nutritional information: 411 calories, 14 percent fat (6.56 grams), 57 percent carbohydrate, 29 percent protein, 5.62 grams fiber

BREAKFAST 16

Fruit 'n' Granola Parfait:

In a tall glass, layer chopped fresh strawberries, nonfat yogurt, honey, low-fat granola, and bananas.

1 cup orange juice

Nutritional information: 481 calories, 6 percent fat (3.31 grams), 84 percent carbohydrate, 10 percent protein, 7.92 grams fiber

BREAKFAST 17

Egg White Omelet:

In a nonstick skillet, sauté ¼ cup sliced mushrooms, ¼ cup chopped asparagus, and ¼ cup onions until tender. Remove from pan, spray pan with vegetable spray, and pour in 3 whipped egg whites. Cook slowly until firm. Remove from pan, fill omelet with mushroom mixture, and fold over. Salt and pepper to taste.

1 slice whole wheat toast topped with 1 teaspoon all-fruit jam

1 cup fresh peaches

Nutritional information: 361 calories, 8 percent fat (3.47 grams), 70 percent carbohydrate, 22 percent protein, 10.8 grams fiber

BREAKFAST 18

Banana-Berry Oatmeal:

In a small pan, heat 1 cup nonfat milk until simmering. Add 1 small chopped banana and ¼ cup chopped berries, stir, then add ½ cup instant oatmeal and 2 tablespoons toasted wheat germ. Simmer for 2 minutes, stirring occasionally, until milk is absorbed. Let stand 2 minutes. Sweeten with honey.

1 cup orange juice

Nutritional information: 512 calories, 7 percent fat (4.3 grams), 79 percent carbohydrate, 14 percent protein, 7.9 grams fiber

LUNCH IDEAS

LUNCH 1

½ chicken sandwich, made from 1 slice whole wheat bread, 2 ounces chicken breast, 1 Ortega green chili (canned), and 1 teaspoon Dijon mustard

1 cup tossed salad made from leaf lettuce and red cabbage with ½ cup mandarin oranges and 2 tablespoons fat-free raspberry vinaigrette dressing

1 cup nonfat milk

Nutritional information: 376 calories, 16 percent fat (6.7 grams), 52 percent carbohydrate, 32 percent protein, 7.2 grams fiber

LUNCH 2

2 slices lean turkey breast

10 fat-free whole wheat crackers

15 baby carrots

½ cup pineapple chunks

1 cup nonfat milk, flavored with nutmeg

Nutritional information: 510 calories, 21 percent fat (12 grams), 49 percent carbohydrate, 30 percent protein, 8.6 grams fiber

LUNCH 3

1 cup vegetable-bean soup (canned), heated with ½ cup frozen carrots and peas

1 whole wheat roll or 1 slice whole wheat bread

1 ounce soy cheese

1 piece of fruit

1 cup nonfat milk

Nutritional information: 509 calories, 22 percent fat (12.7 grams), 55 percent carbohydrate, 23 percent protein, 9.6 grams fiber

LUNCH 4

Vegetable Fajita:

Warm 1 corn tortilla and fill with 1 ounce grated fat-free cheddar cheese or soy cheese, ½ cup cooked fajita-style vegetables with black beans (in frozen-vegetables section of supermarket), ¼ cup black beans, 2 tablespoons salsa

1 cup plain nonfat yogurt mixed with ½ cup strawberries (or any fresh fruit)

1 cup orange juice with a lime twist

Nutritional information: 475 calories, 6 percent fat (3.3 grams), 71 percent carbohydrate, 23 percent protein, 10.2 grams fiber

LUNCH 5

Tossed Mexican Salad:

Mix 2 cups chopped romaine lettuce, ¼ cup diced red cabbage, ¼ cup grated carrot, 1 ounce fat-free cheddar cheese or soy cheese, ⅓ cup canned kidney beans, rinsed and drained, 2 ounces diced chicken breast, ¼ medium avocado, sliced, 2 tablespoons fat-free spicy dressing

1 ounce oven-baked tortilla chips (or make your own by cutting corn tortillas into wedges and baking until crisp)
1 cup nonfat milk

Nutritional information: 584 calories, 33 percent fat (21.5 grams), 38 percent carbohydrate, 29 percent protein, 11.9 grams fiber

LUNCH 6

Shrimp salad, made with 3 ounces cooked small shrimp, 4 cucumber slices, 3 cups chopped mixed greens, 1 large chopped tomato, 3 tablespoons fat-free dressing
1 baked sweet potato topped with 1 teaspoon chopped walnuts
1 cup nonfat milk
1 piece fruit

Nutritional information: 448 calories, 23 percent fat (11.6 grams), 49 percent carbohydrate, 29 percent protein, 7.8 grams fiber

LUNCH 7

Peanut butter sandwich, made with 2 slices whole-grain bread, 2 tablespoons peanut butter, 1 sliced banana or apple

1 cup sliced raw vegetables dunked in 2 tablespoons fat-free sour cream dressing
1 cup nonfat milk

Nutritional information: 617 calories, 28 percent fat (19.5 grams), 56 percent carbohydrate, 16 percent protein, 14.1 grams fiber

LUNCH 8

Chicken salad, made with 3 cups mixed salad greens, 3 ounces chicken breast (cubed and mixed with ¼ cup chopped celery and 2 teaspoons light mayonnaise), 1 large chopped tomato, 2 tablespoons chopped red onion, ¼ cup grated carrots, 1 teaspoon roasted sunflower seeds, 3 tablespoons fat-free dressing

½ fresh papaya drizzled with lime or lemon juice
1 cup nonfat milk or soymilk

Nutritional information: 453 calories, 23 percent fat (11.8 grams), 43 percent carbohydrate, 34 percent protein, 9.9 grams fiber

LUNCH 9

Sweet Potato Chowder,* 1 serving

Tossed salad, made with 2 cups chopped romaine lettuce, ½ cup kidney beans (canned and drained), 2 tablespoons chopped green onions, 1 large tomato cut into ¼-inch wedges, 2 tablespoons vinaigrette salad dressing

2 cups watermelon or 1 piece fruit
1 cup nonfat milk or soymilk

Nutritional information: 492 calories, 16 percent fat (9.0 grams), 63 percent carbohydrate, 21 percent protein, 18.7 grams fiber

LUNCH 10

Bulgur, Pear, and Greens,* 1 serving
Succulent Chicken,* 1 serving

Kiwi and mandarin orange salad, made with 1 kiwi, peeled and sliced, 1 cup canned mandarin oranges, and 1 teaspoon sugared ginger

Nutritional information: 512 calories, 17 percent fat (9.9 grams), 58 percent carbohydrate, 25 percent protein, 14.1 grams fiber

DINNER IDEAS

DINNER 1

Vegetable Poached Salmon,* 1 serving

1 baked potato topped with

> *2 tablespoons fat-free sour cream*

1 cup steamed broccoli

1 cup nonfat milk

Nutritional information: 673 calories, 25 percent fat (18.9 grams), 43 percent carbohydrate, 32 percent protein, 8.3 grams fiber

DINNER 2

With 2 cups spaghetti squash, cooked and peeled, add ¾ cup marinara sauce made with 3 ounces ground turkey breast

1 cup steamed green beans

Salad made with 1 cup spinach, 1 tablespoon diced red onion, 2 tablespoons sliced mushrooms, 2 tablespoons chopped tomato, 1 tablespoon fat-free vinaigrette dressing

1 piece fruit

Water

Nutritional information: 542 calories, 23 percent fat (14.0 grams), 53 percent carbohydrate, 24 percent protein, 19.7 grams fiber

DINNER 3

3 ounces roasted turkey breast

2 cups grilled eggplant and zucchini (2 teaspoons olive oil used in preparation)

1 broiled tomato

½ cup small boiled or roasted potatoes with chives

Carrot-apple salad, made with 1 cup grated carrots, ½ apple, chopped, 1 tablespoon raisins, 1 tablespoon lemon juice, 2 tablespoons low-fat mayonnaise, and salt and pepper to taste

Water

Nutritional information: 640 calories, 30 percent fat (21.5 grams), 50 percent carbohydrate, 20 percent protein, 13.6 grams fiber

DINNER 4

Chicken Fajitas:

Mix 4 tablespoons lime juice and ½ cup chopped cilantro and coat 4 ounces of chicken breast cut into strips. Mix with ¾ cup sliced red and green bell peppers and ¾ cup sliced red onion. Spray non-stick pan with vegetable oil and stir-fry chicken–vegetable mixture until done. Fill two warmed 10-inch whole wheat tortillas and top with 4 tablespoons salsa and 2 tablespoons fat-free sour cream.

Fresh Spinach-Raspberry Salad:

Place 2 cups packaged, pretrimmed spinach in a bowl and top with 2 tablespoons thinly sliced red onion, 3 sliced mushrooms, and 10 fresh raspberries (or ½ sliced fresh peach). Drizzle 2 tablespoons of fat-free raspberry vinaigrette dressing over the top.

1 cup fresh pineapple cubes and mango slices with a pinch of cayenne

Water

Nutritional information: 546 calories, 10 percent fat (6.4 grams), 57 percent carbohydrate, 33 percent protein, 13.7 grams fiber

DINNER 5

Citrus Chicken,* 1 serving

Sautéed Mushrooms:

Wash 10 mushrooms and sauté with 1 teaspoon olive oil, 3 diced cloves of garlic, ¼ cup white wine, and salt and pepper to taste.

Wilted Spinach with Sesame:

In a medium saucepan, heat 3 tablespoons chicken broth and one minced garlic clove. Add 2 cups fresh spinach and sauté only until wilted (about 2 minutes). Add 1 tablespoon soy sauce and 1 teaspoon sesame seeds.

1 medium sweet potato, baked
Sparkling water with a twist of lemon

Nutritional information: 559 calories, 22 percent fat (14 grams), 37 percent carbohydrate, 41 percent protein, 10.5 grams fiber

DINNER 6

Lentil Soup with Root Vegetables,* 1 serving
1 slice whole wheat bread with 1 tablespoon Olive Oil Dip with a Zing*
1 cup steamed carrots
2 sliced tomatoes
Sparkling water with a dash of lime juice

Nutritional information: 569 calories, 25 percent fat (16 grams), 60 percent carbohydrate, 15 percent protein, 21 grams fiber

DINNER 7

Broiled Halibut with Corn Salsa,* 1 serving

½ cup brown rice cooked in chicken broth and mixed with 2 tablespoons slivered almonds

½ baked acorn squash

Tossed salad made with 2 cups mixed greens, ½ sliced winter pear, 2 tablespoons sliced red onion, and 2 tablespoons fat-free vinaigrette dressing.

1 cup nonfat milk

Nutritional information: 668 calories, 15 percent fat (11.0 grams), 59 percent carbohydrate, 26 percent protein, 19.2 grams fiber

Recipes

Appetizers, Snacks, and Lunches

HERBED EGGPLANT CAPONATA

This vegetable compote is good as a topping on whole wheat crackers or bread, as a stuffing for pocket bread, or as a side dish to spaghetti.

> 3 tablespoons olive oil
> 1 medium eggplant, peeled and diced
> 1 medium onion, diced
> 1 medium green pepper, seeded and diced
> 1 stalk celery, diced
> 2 cloves garlic, minced
> 1 14-ounce can diced stewed tomatoes
> ¼ cup slivered almonds
> 2 tablespoons capers, drained
> ¼ teaspoon red pepper flakes
> 1 teaspoon honey
> 1 teaspoon oregano
> ½ teaspoon crushed rosemary

Place oil in large, nonstick skillet, heat, and add first 6 ingredients. Sauté for 10 minutes. Add remaining ingredients, bring to a boil. Reduce heat and simmer for 15 minutes, stirring often. Remove from heat, cool slightly; cover and chill for up to two days. Serve with assorted whole wheat crackers and bread.

Makes 8 servings.

Nutritional information per serving: 116 calories, 54 percent fat (7 grams, 1-plus gram saturated fat), 38 percent carbohydrate, 8 percent protein, 4 grams fiber, 40 milligrams calcium

OLIVE OIL DIP WITH A ZING

Our family has made a meal of whole wheat sourdough or herbed whole wheat bread dipped in this oil, along with a tossed salad (such as the Asian Spinach Salad, page 262).

> 1 cup extra-virgin olive oil
> ½ cup balsamic vinegar
> 1 teaspoon red pepper flakes
> 1 teaspoon minced garlic
> 1 tablespoon finely chopped Italian parsley
> Salt and pepper to taste
> Whole wheat sourdough bread

Mix all ingredients and let stand for 1 hour. Use as dipping oil for whole wheat sourdough or herbed whole wheat bread.

Nutritional information (2 tablespoons oil and 2 slices bread): 376 calories, 68 percent fat (28.5 grams, 3.9 grams saturated fat), 27 percent carbohydrate, 5 percent protein, 1.4 grams fiber, 38 milligrams calcium

THE STONE AGE ZINGER SMOOTHIE

Time is no excuse for not eating lunch when it takes only 5 minutes to make this juice. It's extra high in antioxidants, too!

> 4 carrots, peeled
> 1 stalk celery
> 1 medium apple, quartered and seeded

1 tablespoon sliced fresh ginger

½ red pepper, seeded

Dash of Tabasco sauce

Lemon zest

Juice all ingredients except zest in a juicer. Pour into a tall glass and top with lemon zest.

Makes one 16-ounce serving or

two 8-ounce servings.

Nutritional information for the 16-ounce serving: 225 calories, 4 percent saturated fat (0.2 grams), 89 percent carbohydrate, 7 percent protein, 6.5 grams fiber

GARBANZO CILANTRO DIP

Garbanzos are a filling, hearty topping for crackers, vegetables, or pocket bread. The cilantro gives this dip a clean, refreshing taste.

1 tablespoon olive oil

2 cloves garlic, minced

2 cups diced onion

2 tablespoons raspberry vinegar

1 15½-ounce can garbanzo beans, with
  liquid

3 tablespoons chopped fresh cilantro

½ teaspoon cumin

Salt and pepper to taste

Cilantro sprigs

Heat oil in nonstick skillet over medium heat. Add garlic and onions and sauté until golden brown. Add vinegar and heat until liquid evaporates, approximately 5 minutes. Cool. Drain garbanzo beans and retain liquid. Place onion mixture, beans, cilantro, cumin, half of the bean liquid, and salt and pepper to taste in blender and purée. Pour into a medium serving bowl, garnish with cilantro sprigs, and serve with whole wheat crackers, baked tortilla chips, whole wheat pita bread, or raw vegetables.

Makes 8 ¼-cup servings.

Nutritional information per serving: 96 calories, 22 percent fat (2.3 grams, less than 0.5 grams saturated fat), 65 percent carbohydrate, 13 percent protein, 3.8 grams fiber, 26 milligrams calcium

QUICK 'N' EASY CALICO BEAN CHILI

It takes only 30 minutes to make a pot of this tasty chili, which will last you all week for snacks and quick-fix lunches. It's loaded with fiber, B vitamins (especially folic acid), calcium, magnesium, and iron, too. Serve with cornbread and a tossed salad to turn it into a meal.

2 28-ounce cans crushed tomatoes, drained

1 15-ounce can Great Northern beans, drained

1 15-ounce can pinto or garbanzo beans, drained

2 15-ounce cans black beans, drained

2 tablespoons chili powder

1 teaspoon cumin

1 4.5-ounce can chopped green chilies, undrained

4 tablespoons chopped cilantro

¼ cup nonfat sour cream

In large soup pot, combine all ingredients, except cilantro and sour cream, and mix well. Bring to a boil. Reduce heat to medium. Cover and simmer for 10 to 15 minutes. Serve topped with cilantro and sour cream.

Makes 5 2-cup servings.

Nutritional information per serving: 385 calories, 5 percent fat (2.0 grams, less than 0.5 grams saturated fat), 71 percent carbohydrate, 24 percent protein, 17.6 grams fiber, 185 milligrams calcium

PEACH EGGNOG FRAÎCHE

Need a light and sweet snack? Try this whipped fruit pudding topped with peaches.

> 2 cans peaches canned in own juice,
>   drained
> 1 cup nonfat plain yogurt
> ¼ cup honey
> Dash of nutmeg
> 1 teaspoon rum flavoring (or 2 tablespoons
>   rum)
> 1 envelope gelatin
> 2 tablespoons water
> 4 fresh peaches, peeled and sliced, or 1 can
>   sliced peaches canned in own juice,
>   drained, for garnish

In blender, combine peaches, yogurt, honey, nutmeg, and rum flavoring. Whip until smooth. In small saucepan, combine gelatin and water and heat until gelatin dissolves, approximately 3 minutes. Pour gelatin into blender with peach mixture and whip for 2 minutes until blended. Pour into bowl and chill for 2 hours. When ready to serve, divide fraîche into 4 tall stemmed glasses and top with peach slices.

Makes 4 servings.

Nutritional information per serving: 175 calories, 1 percent fat (less than 0.2 grams, 0 grams saturated fat), 87 percent carbohydrate, 12 percent protein, 1.5 grams fiber, 129 milligrams calcium

Soups

SWEET POTATO CHOWDER

A hearty bowl of this chowder will fill you up without filling you out. It's creamy, colorful, and rich in antioxidants.

2 teaspoons olive oil

½ cup chopped Spanish onion

1½ teaspoons dried thyme

1 bay leaf

½ teaspoon salt

¼ teaspoon ground black pepper

4 cups vegetable broth

3 sweet potatoes or yams (orange flesh),
    peeled and cut into 1-inch cubes

½ cup evaporated skim milk (or soymilk)

½ teaspoon minced fresh garlic

¼ cup chopped fresh parsley

Heat oil in a large stockpot over medium heat. Add onion and sauté 5 minutes, until tender and golden. Add thyme, bay leaf, salt, and pepper and stir to coat onion with herbs. Add broth and sweet potatoes and bring mixture to a boil. Reduce heat, partially cover, and simmer 20 minutes, until potatoes are fork-tender. Remove from heat and stir in milk. Remove bay leaf and transfer one quarter of the mixture to a blender or food processor. Process until smooth. Return purée to the pot and stir in garlic. Ladle chowder into bowls and top with chopped parsley.

Makes 4 2-cup servings.

Nutritional information per serving: 183 calories, 19 percent fat (3.8 grams, less than 1 gram saturated fat), 61 percent carbohydrate, 20 percent protein, 3.15 grams fiber, 138 milligrams calcium

SHRIMP SEVICHE SOUP

This refreshing soup is a great supper for hot summer nights. You get whopping doses of the B vitamins, vitamin C, iron, and selenium for few calories and very little fat. All you need is crusty bread to make a meal.

¾ pound medium shrimp, peeled and
deveined
3 beefsteak tomatoes (about 2 pounds),
halved
½ cup vegetable broth
½ cup tomato juice
2 tablespoons fresh lemon juice
1 garlic clove, peeled
½ teaspoon salt
2 tablespoons chopped fresh cilantro
2 tablespoons chopped fresh parsley

Cook shrimp in a large pot of rapidly boiling water for 3 minutes, until bright red and cooked through. Rinse under cold water to prevent further cooking and set aside.

Dice one of the tomatoes into small pieces and set aside.

In a blender or food processor, combine remaining tomatoes, broth, tomato juice, lemon juice, garlic, and salt. Purée until smooth.

Transfer mixture to a large bowl and stir in shrimp, diced tomatoes, cilantro, and parsley.

Refrigerate 1 hour before serving.

Makes 4 1½-cup servings.

Nutritional information per serving: 145 calories, 11 percent fat (1.8 grams, less than 0.5 grams saturated fat), 34 percent carbohydrate, 55 percent protein, 3.3 grams fiber, 52 milligrams calcium

CHICKEN, BARLEY, AND VEGETABLE SOUP

This soup is a meal in itself. Serve alone or with a salad. It's high in fiber, B vitamins (especially niacin, B_6, and B_{12}), iron, and selenium.

>2 teaspoons olive oil
>1 pound skinless, boneless chicken breasts,
>   cut into 1-inch cubes
>½ cup chopped onion
>2 celery stalks, chopped
>2 carrots, peeled and cut crosswise into rounds
>1½ teaspoons dried oregano
>1 bay leaf
>½ teaspoon salt
>¼ teaspoon ground black pepper
>4 cups nonfat chicken broth
>½ cup uncooked pearl barley
>½ cup frozen green peas
>2 tablespoons vermouth or sherry

Heat oil in a large stockpot over medium heat. Add chicken and brown on all sides. Remove chicken from pan and set aside.

To the same pot, add onion, celery, and carrots and sauté 4 minutes, until tender.

Add oregano, bay leaf, salt, and pepper and stir to coat vegetables with herbs.

Return chicken to pan and add broth and barley. Bring to a boil, reduce heat, partially cover and simmer 1 hour, until barley is tender.

Stir in peas and vermouth or sherry and simmer 2 minutes to heat through.

Remove bay leaf, ladle soup into bowls, and serve hot.

Makes 4 servings.

Nutritional information per serving: 317 calories, 16 percent fat (5.5 grams, 1 gram saturated fat), 39 percent carbohydrate, 45 percent protein, 6.27 grams fiber, 48 milligrams calcium

BUTTERNUT SQUASH SOUP WITH CHIPOTLE PEPPER AND HAZELNUT PEAR CHUTNEY

The delicate flavors give this soup an elegance appropriate for any dinner party, but a simplicity suitable for family dinners.

Soup

1 tablespoon canola oil

1 cup sliced onion

1 teaspoon minced fresh ginger

1 garlic clove, chopped

¼ teaspoon cinnamon

1 butternut squash (about 2 pounds),
  peeled, seeded, and diced

3 cups chicken broth

½ teaspoon dried thyme

¼ cup honey

1 chipotle pepper in adobo sauce, rinsed,
  cleaned of seeds, and chopped

Salt and pepper to taste

Chutney

⅓ cup chopped roasted hazelnuts

2 small pears or 2 small apples, peeled and
  diced

1 tablespoon lemon juice

¼ teaspoon cinnamon

A pinch of cardamom

Chicken broth, optional

Soup: Heat oil in large, heavy pot over medium-low heat. Mix in onion, ginger, garlic, and cinnamon. Sauté, stirring, about 5 minutes, until tender.

Add squash, chicken broth, thyme, and honey. Stir well. Bring to a boil. Reduce heat, cover, and simmer 10 to 15 minutes, until squash is soft.

Remove from heat and cool slightly. Working in small batches, purée soup in blender or food processor until smooth. Return puréed soup to pot. Add chipotle pepper and stir. Season to taste with salt and pepper. Reheat.

Makes 4 2-cup servings.

Chutney: Combine all ingredients. If necessary, thin with chicken broth. Sprinkle 1 tablespoon on top of each bowl of soup before serving.

Nutritional information per serving: 303 calories, 33 percent fat (11 grams, 1 gram saturated fat), 58 percent carbohydrate, 9 percent protein, 6.8 grams fiber, 91 milligrams calcium

CANNELLINI BEAN AND FENNEL SOUP

1 tablespoon olive oil
1 sweet onion, chopped
1 fennel bulb, chopped
2 leeks, chopped (white part only)
1 teaspoon ground thyme
3 cups chicken broth
2 15-ounce cans of cannellini beans,
    drained (reserve ½ cup of beans)
2 garlic cloves, minced
¼ cup grated carrots
1 cup coarsely chopped fresh spinach
Chicken broth (optional)
Fresh chopped parsley
Fat-free Parmesan cheese (optional)
Salt and pepper to taste

In a large saucepan, heat oil over medium–low heat. Add onions, fennel, leeks, and thyme. Cook, stirring occasionally, until vegetables start to caramelize, approximately 10 to 15 minutes. Add chicken broth, all but ½ cup of cannellini beans, garlic, and carrots, and simmer for 10 minutes. Remove from heat, cool slightly. Working in small batches, pour bean–fennel mixture into blender and whip until smooth. Return to pot and add spinach and rest of beans. Heat until spinach wilts and soup is hot. Thin with extra chicken broth, if needed. Serve with parsley and Parmesan. Salt and pepper to taste.

Makes 5 1-cup servings.

Nutritional information per serving: 230 calories, 16 percent fat (4 grams, less than 1 gram saturated fat), 61 percent carbohydrate, 23 percent protein, 6.4 grams fiber, 160 milligrams calcium

LENTIL SOUP WITH ROOT VEGETABLES

A great soup for cold winter days. This recipe makes about 16 cups, which can serve as lunches and snacks throughout the week. A two-cup serving supplies 231 micrograms of folic acid and more than 5 milligrams of iron!

1½ cups dried lentils, washed

2 quarts water

2 tablespoons tomato paste

1 28-ounce can diced tomatoes in own juice

1 baking potato, unpeeled and diced

1 sweet onion, diced

1 leek, white part only, sliced

2 stalks celery, sliced

1 garlic clove, minced

2 carrots, diced

4 mushrooms, sliced

1 tablespoon basil

1 teaspoon salt

1 teaspoon thyme

1 teaspoon oregano

½ teaspoon black pepper

1 10-ounce package frozen chopped spinach

Fat-free Parmesan cheese, optional

Combine all ingredients except spinach in a large heavy soup pot. Cover and simmer for one hour.

During the last 15 minutes, add spinach. To serve, ladle into bowls and sprinkle with fat-free Parmesan cheese, if desired.

Makes 8 2-cup servings.

Nutritional information per serving: 193 calories, 4 percent fat (less than 1 gram, 0 grams saturated fat), 70 percent carbohydrate, 26 percent protein, 8.17 grams fiber, 84 milligrams calcium

HEARTY BARLEY MUSHROOM SOUP

The original comfort food, this rich-tasting soup can double as a meal for lunch or dinner.

1 tablespoon olive oil

1 large yellow onion, finely chopped

2 cloves garlic, minced

1 carrot, peeled and sliced

1 sweet red pepper, chopped

6 shiitake mushrooms, cleaned and sliced

6 button mushrooms, cleaned and sliced

1 cup chopped canned tomatoes

⅓ cup pearl barley

2 cups vegetable broth

½ teaspoon thyme

½ teaspoon rosemary, crumbled

Salt and pepper to taste

In a large, heavy saucepan over medium-low heat, heat oil. Add onion and garlic, cook 5 minutes. Stir in carrot and red pepper, cook until tender, another 5 minutes.

Add the mushrooms and cook, stirring frequently, until tender. Stir in tomatoes and barley. Add broth and seasonings, salt and pepper. Bring to a boil. Reduce heat to low, cover, and simmer until barley is tender (approximately 45 minutes).

Makes 4 1½-cup servings.

Nutritional information per serving: 173 calories, 23 percent fat (4.5 grams, less than 1 gram saturated fat), 62 percent carbohydrate, 15 percent protein, 5.96 grams fiber, 44.5 milligrams calcium

Salads and Dressings

SWEET POTATO 'N' CORN SALAD

It's hard to believe a salad that looks so pretty could taste so good. It's colorful, crunchy, flavorful, rich in antioxidants, and takes only 10 minutes to make. Serve it as a snack, lunch, or side dish.

1 medium sweet potato
½ cup corn, fresh or frozen
¼ cup diced red onion
1 tablespoon balsamic vinegar
1 tablespoon olive oil
1 tablespoon chopped cilantro
Salt and pepper to taste

Microwave sweet potato until cooked, but firm. The potato needs to hold its shape, so don't overcook—approximately 5 to 7 minutes, depending on microwave and size of potato. While potato is cooking, steam corn for 5 minutes or until heated through. Remove potato from microwave, cool slightly, peel, and chop into 1-inch cubes. Combine with other ingredients and mix gently.

Makes 1 serving.

Nutritional information: 318 calories, 39 percent fat (13.7 grams, 2 grams saturated fat), 55 percent carbohydrate, 6 percent protein, 6.5 grams fiber, 45 milligrams calcium

APPLE GRAPE SALAD

Combining fruit with vegetables is a great way to revive your love of salads. This salad is a bit sweet, so is a good accompaniment to chicken (such as Citrus Chicken, pages 265–66).

¼ cup canola oil
¼ cup apple juice (fresh-squeezed is best)
1 tablespoon raspberry vinegar
¼ teaspoon ground cloves
¼ teaspoon ground cinnamon
4 cups leaf lettuce, chopped
3 medium tart apples or 2 large winter
    pears, cored and thinly sliced
1 cup seedless red grapes, halved

Dressing: In a jar or blender, combine oil, apple juice, vinegar, cloves, and cinnamon. Chill.

Salad: Arrange lettuce on 4 plates. Top with apples or pears. Shake dressing and pour over top. Top with grapes.

Makes 4 servings.

Nutritional information per serving: 228 calories, 54 percent fat (13.7 grams, 1 gram saturated fat), 44 percent carbohydrate, 2 percent protein, 3.6 grams fiber, 51 milligrams calcium

AVOCADO ORANGE VINAIGRETTE SALAD

Avocados might be high in calories, but they are low in saturated fats and high in the type of fats on which we evolved. They also add color, creaminess, and a delightful taste to a salad, not to mention that they are rich in B vitamins, vitamins C and E, and most minerals. Mix them with citrus and the combination is heavenly.

Salad

5 cups mixed greens (European blend with
   red cabbage is especially good)
3 navel oranges, peeled and separated
⅓ red onion, thinly sliced
2 avocados, peeled, pitted, and sliced
½ cup jicama, peeled and thinly sliced

Vinaigrette

¼ cup raspberry vinegar
¼ cup orange juice
1 teaspoon orange zest
Juice of one lemon
¼ teaspoon lemon zest
1 tablespoon honey
¼ teaspoon dry mustard
1 tablespoon poppy seeds
1 tablespoon canola oil

Salad: Wash and dry lettuce. Tear into bite-size pieces if needed. Place equal amounts on four salad plates. Top with orange, onion, avocado, and jicama slices.

Dressing: Combine all ingredients in a jar. Cover and shake well. Use on salads as needed.

Makes 4 servings.

Nutritional information per serving, assuming all dressing is used: 302 calories, 55 percent fat (18.5 grams, 2.8 grams saturated fat), 39 percent carbohydrate, 6 percent protein, 7.6 grams fiber, 130 milligrams calcium

ASIAN SPINACH SALAD

This salad gives spinach a face-lift, combining sweet, sour, and peanuts with the crispness of spinach. It's a great accompaniment to any of the salmon dishes in this book, not to mention its hefty amounts of folic acid, iron, magnesium, selenium, and vitamin C.

Dressing

3 tablespoons canola oil

2 tablespoons rice vinegar

1 tablespoon low-sodium soy sauce

1 tablespoon honey

$\frac{1}{4}$ teaspoon minced ginger

Dash red pepper flakes

Salad

2 cups fresh pea pods, washed and
   stemmed

4 cups spinach, washed and torn into large
   pieces

1 11-ounce can mandarin oranges, drained

$\frac{1}{3}$ cup peanuts, ground

Dressing: In a screw-top jar, combine oil, vinegar, soy sauce, honey, ginger, and red pepper flakes. Cover. Shake well. Chill. Shake well before using.

Makes about $\frac{1}{2}$ cup.

Salad: Steam pea pods for 3 minutes. Chill. Divide spinach evenly between four plates. Arrange pea pods on top of spinach. Top with orange slices and peanuts. Use dressing as needed.

Makes 4 servings.

Nutritional information per serving, assuming all dressing is used: 248 calories, 56 percent fat (15.5 grams, 1.6 grams saturated fat), 33 percent carbohydrate, 11 percent protein, 4.8 grams fiber, 102 milligrams calcium

LEMON, PAPAYA, AND WATERCRESS SALAD

This refreshing salad mixes unusual and complementary flavors of sweet with bitter and citrus with celery to awaken your tastebuds. It's a great side dish for chicken or can accompany a sandwich at lunch. Its fresh taste will linger long after the salad is gone.

4 cups watercress leaves, rinsed and
   drained
¼ cup radish sprouts (mixed sprouts will do)
2 large papayas, peeled, seeded, and diced
2 tablespoons thinly sliced red onion
2 tablespoons raspberry vinegar
2 tablespoons fresh lemon juice
1 tablespoon honey
2 teaspoons celery seeds
¼ teaspoon lemon zest
¼ teaspoon orange zest
¼ teaspoon ground coriander
Salt to taste

Mix watercress and sprouts in a wide, shallow bowl and make a well in the middle. Place papaya in the well and top with red onions.

In a jar, mix remaining ingredients. Cover and shake well. Pour over papaya salad and serve.

Makes 4 servings.

Nutritional information per serving: 85 calories, 3 percent fat (less than 0.5 grams, 0 grams saturated fat), 89 percent carbohydrate, 8 percent protein, 4.4 grams fiber, 81 milligrams calcium

Chicken and Turkey Dishes

CHILI-GLAZED CHICKEN

This spicy chicken will fire up your tastebuds. Serve it with Mexican corn, beans and rice, or Green Beans with Shiitake Mushrooms (page 277).

2 tablespoons hot chili paste

3 tablespoons honey

1 tablespoon soy sauce

2 teaspoons minced ginger

2 tablespoons chicken broth

2 tablespoons cilantro, chopped

4 boneless, skinless chicken breasts

Marinade: Combine first six ingredients. Mix well.

Pour marinade over chicken, turn once. (May marinate up to an hour.)

Grill or broil approximately four minutes on each side, until no longer pink inside.

Makes 4 servings.

Nutritional Information per serving: 181 calories, 8 percent fat (1.51 grams, less than 0.5 grams saturated fat), 30 percent carbohydrate, 62 percent protein, less than 1 gram fiber, 15.5 milligrams calcium

HERB-RUBBED CHICKEN

The flavors in this chicken are robust and satisfying. They'll even fill the house with the smells of home cooking. It's an easy, quick-fix dinner that takes only 5 minutes to prepare and another 30–40 minutes until it's on the table. It's especially good with roasted potatoes or vegetables (such as Roasted Lemon Asparagus and Red Peppers (pages 275–76) or the Stuffed Portobello Mushrooms (pages 274–75).

4 boneless, skinless chicken breasts

2 cloves garlic, minced

1 teaspoon finely chopped fresh rosemary

1 teaspoon thyme

1 tablespoon chopped fresh parsley

Salt to taste

¼ teaspoon black pepper

1 tablespoon olive oil

½ cup chicken broth

¼ cup balsamic vinegar

Preheat oven to 400°F.

Rinse and pat dry chicken. Combine garlic, rosemary, thyme, parsley, salt, and pepper in a small bowl. Mix well.

Drizzle chicken with oil, rub with herb mixture.

Pour chicken broth in heavy roasting pan. Place chicken in pan. Bake 20 minutes. Turn chicken, bake another 10 to 20 minutes or until no longer pink in the center.

Pour the balsamic vinegar over the chicken in the pan. Transfer chicken to a plate. Stir leftover liquid in pan and drizzle over chicken.

Makes 4 servings.

Nutritional information per serving: 136 calories, 11 percent fat (1.6 grams, less than 0.5 grams saturated fat), 2 percent carbohydrate, 87 percent protein, less than 1 gram fiber, 18 milligrams calcium

CITRUS CHICKEN

Light and sunny, this chicken is a great, quick-fix dinner. The leftovers can be sliced onto salads and used in pocket sandwiches with watercress and orange slices.

1 tablespoon olive oil

1 teaspoon fresh lemon juice

1 teaspoon fresh lime juice

2 teaspoons fresh orange juice

1½ teaspoons finely chopped fresh
rosemary or 1 teaspoon dried crushed
rosemary

Salt and pepper to taste

4 boneless, skinless chicken breasts or

1 pound turkey breast

Heat oven to 375°F.

Mix all ingredients, except the chicken.

Place chicken/turkey in a shallow roasting pan. Rub mixture on both sides of poultry. Bake uncovered 10 minutes on each side, brushing with marinade when turned. Cook 20–30 minutes, until no longer pink.

Makes 4 servings.

Nutritional information per serving: 162 calories, 28 percent fat (4.8 grams, less than 1 gram saturated fat), 2 percent carbohydrate, 70 percent protein, less than 1 gram fiber, 19 milligrams calcium

SPICY TURKEY STEW

Serve this tasty and filling stew with corn tortillas for a one-pot meal.

1 tablespoon olive oil

1 pound turkey breast, cut into ½- to 1-inch cubes

1 cup chopped yellow sweet onion

1 garlic clove, minced

1 teaspoon cumin

1 teaspoon chili seasoning

1 teaspoon coriander

Salt and black pepper to taste

1 28-ounce can tomatoes, cut up

1 14.5-ounce can diced tomatoes and green chilies (spicy)

1 15-ounce can black beans, rinsed, drained

1 15-ounce can white beans, rinsed, drained

1 4-ounce can green chilies

⅓ cup nonfat sour cream

⅓ cup nonfat grated cheese (any kind)

In a large, heavy soup pot, heat oil, then add turkey, onion, and garlic. Cook over medium heat for 10 minutes until center of turkey is no longer pink.

Add cumin, chili, coriander, salt, and pepper. Cook for one minute. Stir in both cans of tomatoes.

Bring to a boil, then reduce heat. Cover and simmer for 15 minutes, stirring occasionally.

Add beans and green chilies. Heat through. Serve topped with a dollop of sour cream and cheese.

Makes 5 2-cup servings.

Nutritional information per serving: 525 calories, 21 percent fat (12.4 grams, 3 grams saturated fat), 43 percent carbohydrate, 36 percent protein, 11.3 grams fiber, 237 milligrams calcium

SUCCULENT CHICKEN

It's difficult to keep chicken breast tender, but the coating for this chicken succeeds. Serve with brown rice, steamed vegetables, or Whipped Ginger Sweet Potatoes (page 276).

½ cup nonfat sour cream

½ cup nonfat mayonnaise

1 tablespoon fat-free Parmesan cheese

1 tablespoon soy sauce

½ teaspoon curry powder

½ teaspoon dry mustard

4 boneless, skinless chicken breasts

½ cup whole wheat dry bread crumbs

Combine first six ingredients in a bowl; mix well. Coat the chicken with crumbs and then dip in sour cream mixture.

Place in a baking dish and bake at 350°F for 50 minutes, or until chicken is tender.

Makes 4 servings.

Nutritional information per serving: 226 calories, 10 percent fat (2.6 grams, less than 1 gram saturated fat), 33 percent carbohydrate, 57 percent protein, less than 1 gram fiber, 63 milligrams calcium

Seafood Dishes

BROILED HALIBUT WITH CORN SALSA

An easy and tasty meal that takes only 30 minutes to make. Serve with a tossed salad and your favorite whole grain dish.

4 firm tomatoes (Romas are best), chopped
½ small red onion, chopped
½ cup corn kernels (raw, frozen, canned) heated in a nonstick skillet until toasted
2 tablespoons lemon juice
3 tablespoons green chilies, chopped
3 tablespoons chopped cilantro
Salt and pepper
4 fresh halibut steaks
1 teaspoon olive oil
Salt and pepper

In a medium bowl, mix tomatoes, onions, corn, lemon juice, chilies, cilantro, and salt and pepper to taste. Set aside and let flavors blend.

Heat broiler. Wash halibut and pat dry. Rub fish with olive oil and sprinkle with salt and pepper. Place on rack at least 3 inches from heat and broil for 5 to 10 minutes per side, depending on thickness of fish. Place halibut on plates and top with salsa.

Makes 4 servings.

Nutritional information per serving: 187 calories, 21 percent fat (4.4 grams, 0.5 grams omega-3 fatty acids), 25 percent carbohydrate, 54 percent protein, 2.67 grams fiber, 66.6 milligrams calcium

SHELLFISH STEW

Filling and flavorful for only 254 calories, this stew is good all year-round. Serve with a tossed salad and whole wheat bread. It's super high in B vitamins and minerals, such as selenium and iron, and potassium.

2 tablespoons olive oil

1 cup chopped yellow sweet onion

1 tablespoon minced garlic

1 leek, sliced, white part only

3 teaspoons dried oregano

2 teaspoons dried basil

2 teaspoons fennel seeds

$\frac{1}{4}$ teaspoon hot chili pepper flakes (may use crushed red pepper or crushed chipotle chili pepper flakes)

1 28-ounce can crushed tomatoes with added purée

1 8-ounce bottle clam juice

1 cup V8 juice

2 6$\frac{1}{2}$-ounce cans chopped clams (reserve liquid)

1 pound uncooked medium or large shrimp, peeled and deveined

1 6-ounce can crabmeat, drained

$\frac{1}{4}$ cup fresh chopped parsley

Salt and pepper to taste

Heat olive oil in large, heavy soup pot over medium–low heat. Add onion, garlic, leek, oregano, basil, fennel seeds, and hot chili pepper flakes. Sauté until onion is tender. Add tomatoes, clam juice, and V8 juice and increase heat. Boil gently for 15 minutes. Add clams and liquid, shrimp, and crabmeat. Reduce heat and simmer for 4 minutes, or until shrimp is opaque (be careful not to overcook). Sprinkle the stew with fresh parsley and serve. Season with salt and pepper.

Makes 5 2-cup servings.

Nutritional information per serving: 254 calories, 27 percent fat (7.7 grams, 1 gram saturated fat), 29 percent carbohydrate, 44 percent protein, 3.5 grams fiber, 169 milligrams calcium

HALIBUT STEAKS WITH TOMATOES AND CAPERS

An easy dish filled with flavor. The ginger wakes up your tastebuds, and the capers give this dish a salty bite.

> 3 fresh tomatoes, chopped
> 2 tablespoons chopped fresh basil
> 2 tablespoons capers with 1 teaspoon caper juice
> 1 teaspoon minced fresh ginger
> 2 tablespoons lemon juice
> 2 tablespoons olive oil
> 4 halibut steaks, fresh or frozen
> Salt and pepper to taste

Preheat oven to 425°F.

Whisk first six ingredients together. Let stand at room temperature.

Arrange halibut on a baking sheet. Brush halibut with one quarter of the tomato/caper mix. Season with salt and pepper if desired. Roast until cooked through, about 10 minutes. Transfer fish to plates.

Top halibut with the rest of tomato and caper mix.

Makes 4 servings.

Nutritional information per serving: 280 calories, 35 percent fat (11 grams, 1.5 grams saturated fat), 9 percent carbohydrate, 56 percent protein, 1.3 grams fiber, 92 milligrams calcium

CREAMY DILL SALMON

Looking for a new taste in salmon? The combination of sour cream and dill is sure to please and provides a tender dish that is quick and easy.

> 1 cup nonfat sour cream
> 2 tablespoons Dijon mustard
> 1 teaspoon dried dill
> Nonstick vegetable spray
> 2 pounds salmon fillet
> Salt and pepper to taste
> ½ fresh lemon

Stir together sour cream, mustard, and dill. Leave out at room temperature for 30 minutes.

Preheat oven to 425°F. Lightly spray aluminum foil with nonstick cooking spray. Place salmon on prepared foil, and add salt and pepper to taste. Squeeze fresh lemon over salmon.

Spread with ¼ cup of sauce mixture. Fold foil to enclose salmon, and bake until salmon is opaque, approximately 15 to 25 minutes, depending on thickness of fish. Open foil the last 3 minutes to brown the top of the salmon. Serve with remaining sauce.

Makes 4 servings.

Nutritional information per serving: 366 calories, 36 percent fat (14.8 grams, 3.94 grams omega-3 fatty acids), 9 percent carbohydrate, 55 percent protein, less than 0.5 grams fiber, 36 milligrams calcium

VEGETABLE-POACHED SALMON

The subtle blend of flavors from the vegetables complement, without detracting from, the salmon. One serving supplies almost 2 grams of omega-3 fatty acids.

> 3 cups water
> 1 small onion, thinly sliced
> 1 small leek, thinly sliced

1 small stalk celery, thinly sliced

½ lemon, thinly sliced

1 small carrot, thinly sliced

½ lime, thinly sliced

1 tablespoon chopped fresh parsley

1 bay leaf

10 peppercorns

½ teaspoon salt

¼ teaspoon thyme

4 salmon steaks, 1 to 2 inches thick

½ lemon, thinly sliced, for garnish

½ lime, thinly sliced, for garnish

Combine all above ingredients except salmon and remaining lemon and lime in a large skillet.

Cover and simmer for 15 minutes.

Set salmon in simmering broth, cover, and gently simmer for 10 minutes, or until fish is opaque.

Place on serving plate with fresh lemon and lime garnish. Good served warm or cold.

Makes 4 servings.

Nutritional information per serving: 189 calories, 35 percent fat (7 grams, 1.99 grams omega-3 fatty acids), 15 percent carbohydrate, 50 percent protein, 1.66 grams fiber, 40 milligrams calcium

GINGER BARBECUED SALMON

Salmon doesn't get any easier than this. In the winter, you can broil instead of grilling. Especially good served with Green Beans with Shiitake Mushrooms (page 277).

¼ cup soy sauce

½ teaspoon Worcestershire sauce

½ teaspoon minced fresh ginger

½ teaspoon garlic powder

Nonstick vegetable spray (optional)

1 pound fresh salmon

Mix soy sauce, Worcestershire, ginger, and garlic in a small bowl.

Place salmon skin side down on heated grill. (You may need to use nonstick spray for the grill.)

Baste salmon frequently with soy sauce mixture while cooking.

Cook until salmon changes color to a light pink. Turn over and peel off skin. Continue to baste frequently. Salmon is done when it starts to look opaque, approximately 15 to 20 minutes.

Makes 4 servings.

Nutritional information per serving: 127 calories, 38 percent fat (5.4 grams, 1.5 grams omega-3 fatty acids), 4 percent carbohydrate, 58 percent protein, less than 1 gram fiber, 13 milligrams calcium

CRUSTY BASIL SALMON

This is one of the best salmon dishes I've ever tasted! It might take a little longer to prepare compared to the other salmon recipes, but believe me, it's worth it. You can make the basil sauce the night before and refrigerate it to save preparation time. Keep side dishes mild so this dish can shine.

3 slices whole wheat bread, dried

¼ cup toasted wheat germ

1½ tablespoons pine nuts

2 garlic cloves, minced

Salt and pepper to taste

5 cups fresh basil leaves

⅓ cup olive oil

Nonstick vegetable spray

1 pound boneless salmon fillet

In a food processor or blender, reduce bread to crumbs. Add wheat germ and mix. Remove about ½ cup of the crumb mixture and set aside. Add pine nuts, garlic, salt, and pepper to the processor and blend. Add basil and olive oil in small batches and continue to process until mixture is a thick paste.

Heat oven to 400°F. Spray baking sheet with vegetable spray. Cut salmon fillet into four equal strips and place on baking sheet. Cover the top of each fillet with ¼ of basil mixture. Sprinkle with remaining crumb/wheat germ mixture and bake until salmon begins to look opaque and basil topping is lightly toasted, approximately 10 to 15 minutes, depending on thickness of salmon.

Makes 4 servings.

Nutritional information per serving: 445 calories, 58 percent fat (29 grams, 2.3 grams omega-3 fatty acids), 16 percent carbohydrate, 26 percent protein, 4.3 grams fiber, 121 milligrams calcium

Vegetables

STUFFED PORTOBELLO MUSHROOMS

These mushrooms are a meal in themselves! You can also serve them with chicken, wild game, or salmon. They're rich in niacin, iron, and selenium.

> 4 5- to 6-inch diameter portobello mushrooms, stemmed
> 2 tablespoons olive oil
> 2 tablespoons balsamic vinegar
> 1 teaspoon finely chopped fresh rosemary
> 1 teaspoon thyme
> ½ teaspoon cumin
> 2 garlic cloves, minced
> 1 medium eggplant, peeled and sliced into 1-inch rounds
> 1 teaspoon tahini (roasted sesame seed paste)

Recipes

1 tablespoon fresh lemon juice
Salt and pepper to taste
4 teaspoons fat-free Parmesan cheese

Arrange mushrooms rounded side down on a baking sheet. Put aside.

Preheat oven to 400°F.

In a bowl, whisk together oil, vinegar, rosemary, thyme, cumin, and garlic. Brush both sides of eggplant slices with marinade.

Place eggplant on baking sheet and bake until golden brown, turning once, approximately 5 minutes on each side. Let eggplant cool.

In a food processor or blender, add eggplant, tahini, lemon juice, salt, and pepper. Process until barely smooth.

Spoon mixture evenly into mushroom caps. Sprinkle with Parmesan cheese. Cover with aluminum foil and bake for 15 minutes. Remove foil and continue baking until mushrooms are tender when pierced with a sharp knife, about 10 minutes more. Serve immediately.

Makes 4 servings.

Nutritional information per serving: 141 calories, 49 percent fat (7.7 grams, 1 gram saturated fat), 40 percent carbohydrate, 11 percent protein, 6.0 grams fiber, 35 milligrams calcium

ROASTED LEMON ASPARAGUS AND RED PEPPERS

The lemon brings out the fresh taste of the asparagus, and the red peppers are just pretty. A great accompaniment to any fish or chicken dish. This dish is especially high in folic acid, vitamin C, selenium, and phytochemicals.

4 tablespoons fresh lemon juice
1 tablespoon olive oil
1 teaspoon grated lemon peel
1 pound fresh asparagus spears, washed
    and tough stems removed

Salt and pepper to taste

2 tablespoons roasted red peppers from jar,
chopped

Preheat oven to 400°F.

Mix lemon juice, oil, and lemon peel in large glass baking dish. Add asparagus. Turn to coat. Add salt and pepper, if desired.

Roast asparagus until tender and crisp, approximately 20 minutes, turning occasionally.

Before serving, sprinkle with chopped roasted red peppers.

Makes 4 servings.

Nutritional information per serving: 57 calories, 50 percent fat (3.15 grams, less than 1 gram saturated fat), 34 percent carbohydrate, 16 percent protein, 2.02 grams fiber, 25 milligrams calcium

WHIPPED GINGER SWEET POTATOES

This dish is so simple, yet so tasty. A great side dish for halibut, salmon, or chicken, it is also high in antioxidants.

3 sweet potatoes, peeled and cut into 1-inch
chunks

2 tablespoons minced fresh ginger

2 tablespoons honey

¼ cup chicken broth

Salt and pepper to taste

Steam sweet potatoes until tender, approximately 15 to 20 minutes. Place in a large bowl and add remaining ingredients. With electric mixer, whip until ingredients are light and thoroughly blended. Season with salt and pepper.

Makes 8 ½-cup servings.

Nutritional information per serving: 79 calories, 2 percent fat (less than 1 gram, 0 grams saturated fat), 92 percent carbohydrate, 6 percent protein, 1.76 grams fiber, 13 milligrams calcium

GREEN BEANS WITH SHIITAKE MUSHROOMS

You won't believe these are green beans! If you can't find shiitake, use regular mushrooms. Try this with the Ginger Barbecued Salmon (pages 272–73) or the Chili-Glazed Chicken (page 264).

> 1 pound fresh green beans, rinsed, stemmed
> ¼ cup chicken broth
> 8 shiitake mushrooms, thinly sliced
> ⅓ cup oyster sauce
> ¼ teaspoon red pepper flakes
> 1 teaspoon minced fresh ginger
> 1 teaspoon minced garlic
> ¼ cup chopped cilantro
> 1 teaspoon sesame oil

Steam green beans until tender-crisp. Rinse in cold water to stop cooking and set aside. In a large skillet, heat chicken broth. Add mushrooms and cook for 2 to 3 minutes over medium heat. Remove from heat.

In a small bowl, combine oyster sauce, red pepper flakes, ginger, garlic, and cilantro. Mix well. Add green beans to mushrooms in skillet and return to heat. Pour oil over vegetables, stirring gently to coat evenly. Add oyster-sauce mixture. Continue to heat and stir for 5 minutes.

Makes 6 servings.

Nutritional information per serving: 64 calories, 28 percent fat (2.0 grams, 0.5 grams saturated fat), 56 percent carbohydrate, 16 percent protein, 3.35 grams fiber, 40 milligrams calcium

BUTTERNUT SQUASH AND LEEK CASSEROLE

This casserole is a nice change from typical candied recipes for squash. It's a good accompaniment to any chicken dish.

1 large butternut squash (approximately
  1½ pounds), peeled, seeded, and cut
  into 1-inch cubes
4 tablespoons chicken broth
3 large leeks, white portion only, sliced thin
¾ cup chopped green onion
¼ teaspoon ground nutmeg
Salt and pepper to taste
1 large egg, beaten, or 1½ cups egg substitute
Dash of nutmeg

Heat oven to 350°F. Steam squash until tender (approximately 15 minutes). While squash is steaming, heat chicken broth in a large nonstick skillet, add leeks and onions, and sauté until vegetables are tender, about 5 minutes. Remove from heat. Mash squash with a fork and add nutmeg, salt and pepper, and egg. Add squash mixture to leeks and mix well. Spread in a shallow 2-quart baking dish, sprinkle with nutmeg, and bake for 50 minutes, or until top is lightly browned.

Makes 4 servings.

Nutritional information per serving: 143 calories, 10 percent fat (1.6 grams, less than 1 gram saturated fat), 78 percent carbohydrate, 12 percent protein, 7 grams fiber, 138 milligrams calcium

Recipes

Dishes with Grains:
From Rice and Tortillas to Bread and Oats

BULGUR, PEAR, AND GREENS

A sweet and fruity version of tabbouleh, this salad is rich in antioxidants and fiber.

1 cup dry bulgur

½ cup chopped fresh parsley

2 cloves garlic, minced

4 tablespoons lemon juice

2 teaspoons olive oil

1 teaspoon salt

2 teaspoons pepper

2 teaspoons mustard

2 teaspoons red wine vinegar

4 teaspoons orange juice

2 pears

8 cups arugula, watercress, or other greens

Cook bulgur according to package directions. Let cool. In a large bowl, blend bulgur, parsley, garlic, lemon juice, olive oil, salt and pepper, and mustard. In a small bowl, blend vinegar and orange juice. Cut pears into thin strips and douse with vinegar mixture. Place greens on a plate and top with bulgur mixture, then with marinated sliced pears.

Makes 4 servings, approximately 2½ cups each.

Nutritional information per serving: 222 calories, 13 percent fat (3 grams, less than 0.5 grams saturated fat), 75 percent carbohydrate, 12 percent protein, 11.6 grams fiber, 111 milligrams calcium

WILD RICE GARDEN SALAD

The rich taste and texture of wild rice give this salad a hearty flavor. Great as a side dish or salad for lunch, dinner, or a snack.

3 cups chicken broth
1¼ cups wild rice, washed
1 8½-ounce can water-packed artichokes,
  drained and diced
1¼ pounds firm tomatoes, diced
1 red bell pepper, seeded and diced
¾ cup chopped fresh parsley
3 tablespoons capers, drained
2 teaspoons grated lemon peel
3 tablespoons fresh lemon juice
1 tablespoon honey
Salt and pepper to taste

In a saucepan, heat chicken broth to a boil. Add rice, cover, reduce heat, and simmer until tender, approximately 40 minutes. Place in large bowl, add artichokes, mix, and set aside until cool.

In a separate bowl, mix remaining ingredients. Stir into cooled rice mixture, and add salt and pepper to taste. Serve cool or chilled.

Makes 8 servings.

Nutritional information per serving: 120 calories, 5 percent fat (less than 1 gram, less than 0.1 grams saturated fat), 80 percent carbohydrate, 15 percent protein, 4.6 grams fiber, 20 milligrams calcium

LENTIL AND ORZO SALAD
WITH BELL PEPPERS AND FRESH HERBS

A meal-in-one salad, this dish can be made ahead and used for quick-fix lunches and snacks throughout the week. You'll find the whole-grain orzo at a health food store.

1 cup lentils, rinsed and picked over to
   remove any debris
12 ounces uncooked whole-grain orzo
   (rice-shaped pasta)
1/2 cup balsamic vinegar
2 tablespoons olive oil
1 carrot, peeled and diced
3 roasted red peppers (bottled in water), drained and diced
1 yellow bell pepper, seeded and diced
1 green bell pepper, seeded and diced
1/2 medium red onion, minced
1/3 cup (packed) chopped fresh basil leaves
1/3 cup (packed) chopped fresh cilantro leaves
Salt and black pepper to taste

Place lentils in a medium saucepan and pour over enough cold water to cover. Bring to a boil, reduce heat, and simmer 25 to 30 minutes, until lentils are tender. Drain and transfer lentils to a large bowl.

Cook orzo according to package directions, drain, and add to lentils. Add balsamic vinegar and olive oil and mix well. Add remaining ingredients and toss to combine.

Serve warm or chilled.

Makes 6 1 1/2-cup servings.

Nutritional information per serving: 314 calories, 15 percent fat (5.5 grams, less than 1 gram saturated fat), 66 percent carbohydrate, 19 percent protein, 8.55 grams fiber, 49 milligrams calcium

CRAB AND ARTICHOKE QUESADILLAS WITH FRESH TOMATO SALSA

These quesadillas are great for appetizers, snacks, or a quick lunch. Fresh crab tastes better than canned, but either will do. Each serving is high in selenium, iron, zinc, and B vitamins.

Quesadillas

1 14-ounce can artichoke hearts, drained and chopped

1 cup nonfat ricotta cheese

½ cup grated nonfat mozzarella cheese

¼ cup chopped fresh cilantro

¼ teaspoon salt

¼ teaspoon cayenne pepper

1 cup lump crabmeat, or one 6-ounce can, drained

12 6-inch whole wheat tortillas

Nonstick cooking spray

Fresh Tomato Salsa

2 ripe beefsteak tomatoes, seeded and diced

2 tablespoons minced red onion

2 tablespoons chopped fresh cilantro

2 tablespoons fresh lime juice

2 canned green chilies, minced

Preheat oven to 350°F.

Quesadillas: In a large bowl, combine artichoke hearts, ricotta, mozzarella, cilantro, salt, and cayenne pepper. Mix well. Gently fold in crabmeat.

Spoon mixture evenly onto the centers of 6 tortillas, leaving a quarter-inch border around the edges. Top with second tortilla and press down gently.

Arrange quesadillas on a baking sheet that has been coated with nonstick spray. Cover with foil and bake 20 minutes.

Salsa: Combine all ingredients in a medium bowl. Toss to combine. Cover with plastic and refrigerate until ready to serve.

Slice each quesadilla into wedges and serve with salsa.

Makes 6 servings.

Nutritional information per serving: 249 calories, 8 percent fat (2.6 grams, less than 1 gram saturated fat), 67 percent carbohydrate, 25 percent protein, 8.18 grams fiber, 111 milligrams calcium

SPICY TOFU AND BLACK BEAN CASSEROLE

This dish will become a regular at your house! Even the kids will love it. Make extra tofu filling to make burritos that store well in the refrigerator for quick snacks or lunches later in the week. All that taste and high in folic acid, fiber, B vitamins, vitamin C, calcium, iron (more than 8.7 milligrams per serving!), selenium, and zinc, too.

1 tablespoon olive oil

2 cups chopped yellow onion

1½ cups chopped green sweet peppers

2 cloves garlic, minced

2 teaspoons cumin

1 teaspoon turmeric

1 teaspoon chili powder

¼ teaspoon red pepper flakes

12 ounces firm tofu, crumbled

2 14.5-ounce cans diced tomatoes and green chilies

1 cup picante sauce

1 4-ounce can diced green chilies

2 15-ounce cans black beans, drained

⅓ cup chopped cilantro

12 6-inch corn tortillas

2 cups nonfat cheddar or Monterey Jack cheese

2 cups shredded lettuce

2 medium tomatoes, chopped

½ cup chopped green onions (optional)

¼ cup chopped olives (optional)

½ cup nonfat sour cream

Heat oil in large nonstick soup pot over medium–low heat. Add onion and peppers, sauté for 5 minutes. Add garlic, cumin, turmeric, chili powder, and pepper flakes; cook for 1 minute. Add crumbled tofu and cook for one minute longer.

Next, add tomatoes, picante sauce, green chilies, and black beans. Increase heat, bring to boil, then reduce heat and simmer uncovered for 10 to 15 minutes. Add chopped cilantro.

Preheat oven to 350°F. Spread one-third of the bean mixture over the bottom of a 13 × 9 × 2–inch baking dish. Top with half of the tortillas, overlapping as necessary, and half of the cheese. Add another third of the bean mix, the remaining tortillas, and then another layer of bean mix.

Cover and bake for 40 to 45 minutes, or until heated through.

Sprinkle with remaining cheese. Let stand for 10 minutes.

Top with lettuce and tomato and green onion and olives, if desired.

Cut in squares. Serve with sour cream.

Makes 8 servings.

Nutritional information per serving: 478 calories, 22 percent fat (12 grams, 4 grams saturated fat), 54 percent carbohydrate, 24 percent protein, 12.4 grams fiber, 459 milligrams calcium

TOFU CONFETTI BURRITOS

I cook the tofu and the cabbage mixture and keep them in the refrigerator to make burrito lunches throughout the week. Also good for a quick-fix dinner served with Mexican corn, salad, and fruit.

> 1 tablespoon olive oil
> 16 ounces firm tofu, cut into ¼-inch cubes
> 3 garlic cloves, minced
> 3 tablespoons diced canned green chilies
> 1 tablespoon minced fresh ginger
> 1 small head red cabbage, tough white parts
>   removed, cut into 2-inch-long thin strips
> 2 tablespoons rice vinegar
> 2 tablespoons low-sodium soy sauce

½ cup chopped fresh cilantro

6 whole wheat tortillas

¼ cup grated carrot

Heat oil in large nonstick skillet over medium-high heat. Add tofu cubes and sauté until golden, stirring frequently. Remove from pan and set aside. Add garlic, chilies, and ginger to skillet and stir over medium heat for 30 seconds. Add cabbage and stir-fry until wilted, about 3 minutes. Add vinegar and soy sauce. Continue to stir-fry until cabbage is tender-crisp. Remove from heat, stir in cilantro, and allow mixture to cool slightly.

Place tortillas on a hot griddle until heated through. Divide slaw mixture into 6 equal amounts and spread down center of each tortilla. Top with grated carrot and tofu chunks. Roll into burritos. Slice each burrito in half and serve.

Makes 6 burritos.

Nutritional information per serving: 236 calories, 31 percent fat (8.1 grams, 1 gram saturated fat), 45 percent carbohydrate, 24 percent protein, 4.15 grams fiber, 223 milligrams calcium

CRANBERRY-OAT QUICK BREAD

Top this bread with all-fruit jam, apple butter, peanut butter, or soy butter for breakfast or a snack. It's also good toasted. Don't overbake, or it will be dry.

2½ cups whole wheat flour

¾ cup rolled oats (regular or quick cooking)

2 teaspoons baking powder

1 teaspoon baking soda

¼ teaspoon salt

1½ cups nonfat vanilla yogurt

½ cup honey

2 egg whites

2 teaspoons vanilla extract

1 cup dried cranberries

Nonstick cooking spray

Preheat oven to 350°F.

In a large bowl, combine flour, oats, baking powder, baking soda, and salt. Mix well with a fork, make a well in the center, and set aside.

Whisk together yogurt, honey, egg whites, and vanilla. Pour into well in dry ingredients and fold until just blended. Fold in cranberries. Pour batter into an 8-inch loaf pan that has been coated with nonstick spray.

Bake 1 hour, until a knife inserted near the center comes out clean. Cool in pan, on a wire rack, for 10 minutes. Remove bread from pan and cool completely.

Makes 1 loaf (10 servings).

Nutritional information per serving: 248 calories, 4 percent fat (1 gram, less than 0.5 grams saturated fat), 83 percent carbohydrate, 13 percent protein, 5.28 grams fiber, 91 milligrams calcium

MAPLE BAKED APPLES
WITH TOASTED OATS AND ALMONDS

Tart apples work best for this recipe—their slightly sour taste pairs well with the sweet maple syrup and nutty almond flavor. You can also substitute firm peaches for the apples, if desired.

4 Granny Smith apples (about 2 pounds),

   peeled, cored, and sliced

6 tablespoons maple syrup, divided

¾ teaspoon cinnamon

¼ teaspoon ground nutmeg

½ cup rolled oats

½ cup sliced almonds

2 tablespoons whole wheat flour

Preheat oven to 400°F.

Combine apples and 2 tablespoons of the maple syrup in a large nonstick skillet over medium-high heat. Sauté until apples are tender, about 10 minutes. Transfer apples to a 9-inch pie plate and set aside.

In a small bowl, whisk together remaining 4 tablespoons maple syrup, cinnamon, and nutmeg. Add oats, almonds, and flour and mix well. Spread mixture over apple slices.

Bake 40 minutes, until top is golden brown. Cool slightly before serving.

Makes 4 2/3-cup servings.

Nutritional information per serving: 355 calories, 25 percent fat (10 grams, 1 gram saturated fat), 69 percent carbohydrate, 6 percent protein, 7.85 grams fiber, 86 milligrams calcium

Sources of Wild Game

Broken Arrow Ranch, Ingram, Texas (800)962-GAME.
   www.brokenarrowranch.com
Gourmet Bison Company, Red Field, South Dakota (888)72-BISON.
   www.gourmetbison.com
Hills Foods, Inc., Brunaby, British Columbia (604)421-3100. *www.hillsfoods.com*
Johnson Emu, Inc., Eva, Alabama (256)796-6353. *www.johnsonemu.com*

Suggested Reading

Allman W: *The Stone Age Present*. New York, Simon & Schuster, 1994.

Allport S: *The Primal Feast: Food, Sex, Foraging, and Love*. New York, Harmony Books, 2000.

Boaz N: *Eco Homo*. New York, Basic Books, 1997.

Buss D: *Evolutionary Psychology: The New Science of the Mind*. Boston, Allyn and Bacon, 1999.

Crawford M, Marsh D: *Nutrition and Evolution*. New Caanan, Conn., Keats Publishing, Inc., 1995.

Eaton S, Shostak M, Konner M: *The Paleolithic Prescription*. New York, Harper & Row, 1988.

Kingdon J: *Self-Made Man*. New York, John Wiley & Sons, 1993.

Lewin R: *The Origin of Modern Humans*. New York, Scientific American Library, 1993 and 1998.

Nesse R, Williams G: *Why We Get Sick*. New York, Vintage Books, 1994.

Simopoulos A: *Evolutionary Aspects of Nutrition and Health: Diet, Exercise, Genetics, and Chronic Disease*. Basel, Karger, 1999.

Stearns S: *Evolution in Health and Disease*. New York, Oxford University Press, 1999.

Tattersall I: *Becoming Human*. New York, Harcourt Brace & Company, 1998.

Trevathan W, Smith E, McKenna J: *Evolutionary Medicine*. New York, Oxford University Press, 1999.

Tudge C: *The Time Before History*. New York, Simon & Schuster, 1996.

Selected References

Chapter 1

Andrews P, Martin L: Hominid dietary evolution. *Phil Tr R Soc L* 1991;334:199–209.

Armelagos G: The rival superhighway. *The Sciences* 1998; Jan/Feb: 24–29.

Bogin B: From caveman cuisine to fast food: The evolution of human nutrition. *Gr Horm & IGF R* 1998;8:79–86.

Collinson M, Hooker J: Fossil evidence of interactions between plants and plant-eating mammals: *Phil Tr R Soc L* 1991;333:197–208.

Eaton S, Eaton S, Sinclair A, et al: Dietary intake of long-chain polyunsaturated fatty acids during the paleolithic. *World Rev N* 1998;83:12–23.

Eaton S, Konner M, Shostak M: Stone agers in the fast lane: Chronic degenerative diseases in evolutionary perspective. *Am J Med* 1998;84:739–749.

Flannery K: The origins of agriculture. *Ann R Anthr* 1973;2:271–310.

Galef B: Food selection: Problems in understanding how we choose foods to eat. *Neurosci B* 1996;20:67–73.

Grigg D: The geography of food consumption: A review. *Prog H Geog* 1995;19:338–354.

Harris B: Growing taller, living longer? Anthropometric history and the future of old age. *Ageing Soc* 1997;17:491–512.

Henry C: New food processing technologies: From foraging to farming to food technology. *P Nutr Soc* 1997;56:855–863.

Klein R: The archeology of modern human origins. *Evol Anthr* 1992;1:5–14.

Kuttner R: Paleolithic nutrition. *N Eng J Med* 1985;May 30:1458–1459.

Leonard W, Robertson M: Comparative primate energetics and hominid evolution. *Am J P Anth* 1997;102;265–281.

Leonard W, Robertson M: Evolutionary perspectives on human nutrition: The influence of brain and body size on diet and metabolism. *Am J Hum B* 1994;6:77–88.

Leonard W, Robertson M: Nutritional requirements and human evolution: A bioenergetics model. *Am J Hum B* 1992;4:179–195.

Macko S, Engel M, Andrusevich V, et al: Documenting the diet in ancient human populations through stable isotope analysis of hair. *Phil Tr R Soc L* 1999;354:66–75.

Milton K: A hypothesis to explain the role of meat-eating in human evolution. *Evol Anthro* 1999;8:11–21.

Ministry of Agriculture, Fisheries and Foods: Household food consumption and expenditure, 1990. With a study of trends over the period 1940–1990. London, HMSO, 1995.

Ogilvie M, Curran B, Trinkaus E: Incidence and patterning of dental enamel hypoplasia among the Neanderthals. *Am J P Anth* 1989;79:25–41.

Peters C, O'Brien E: The early hominid plant-food niche: Insights from an analysis of plant exploitation by Homo, Pan, and Papio in Eastern and Southern Africa. *Curr Anthr* 1981;22:127–140.

Schurr M, Powell M: Changes in infant nutrition with the evolution of food-production: Isotopic evidence from the North-American midcontinent. *Am J P Anth*, 1999;S28:244–245.

Smith B: Patterns of molar wear in hunter-gatherers and agriculturalists. *Am J P Anth* 1984;63:39–56.

Speth J: Early hominid hunting and scavenging: The role of meat as an energy source. *J Hum Evol* 1989;18:329–343.

Sponheimer M, Lee-Thorp J: Isotopic evidence for the diet of an early hominid, Australopithecus africanus. *Science* 1999;283:368–370.

Stahl A: Hominid dietary selection before fire. *Curr Anthr* 1984;25:151–168.

Swisher C, Curtis G, Jacob T, et al: Age of the earliest known hominids in Java, Indonesia. *Science* 1994;263:1118–1121.

Vogel G: Did early African hominids eat meat? *Science* 1999;283:303.

von Koenigswald W, Rensberger J, Pretzschner H: Changes in the tooth enamel of early Paleocene mammals allowing increased diet diversity. *Nature* 1987;328:150–152.

Widdowson E: Contemporary human diets and their relation to health and growth: Overview and conclusions. *Phil Tr R Soc L* 1991;334:289–295.

Wrongham R, Jones J, Laden G, et al: The raw and the stolen: Cooking and the ecology of human origins. *Curr Anthro* 1999;40:567–594.

Chapter 2

Albertson A, Tobelmann R: Consumption of grain and whole-grain foods by an American population during the years 1990 to 1992. *J Am Diet A* 1995;95:703–704.

Andlauer W, Furst P: Antioxidative power of phytochemicals with special reference to cereal. *Cereal F M* 1998;43:356–360.

Brand J, Cherikoff V, Truswell A: The nutritional composition of Australian Aboriginal bushfoods. 3. Seeds and nuts. *Fd Tech Aust* 1985;37:275–279.

Broadhurst C, Cunnane S, Crawford M: Rift Valley lake fish and shellfish provided brain-specific nutrition for early Homo. *Br J Nutr* 1998;79:3–21.

Bruemmer B, White E, Vaughan T, et al: Fluid intake and the incidence of bladder cancer among middle-aged men and women in a three-county area of western Washington. *Nutr Cancer* 1997;29:163–168.

Cachel S: Dietary shifts and the European Upper Paleolithic transition. *Curr Anthr* 1997;38:579–603.

Crawford M, Bloom M, Broadhurst C, et al: Evidence for the unique function of docosahexaenoic acid during the evolution of the modern hominid brain. *Lipids* 1999;34:S39–S47.

Danielson D, Reinhard K: Human dental microwear caused by calcium oxalate phytoliths in prehistoric diet of the Lower Pecos Region, Texas. *Am J P Anth* 1998; 107:297–304.

Eaton S: Humans, Lipids, and evolution. *Lipids* 1992;27:814–820.

Eaton S: Fiber intake in prehistoric times, in Leeds A R (ed): *Dietary Fibre Perspectives Review and Bibliography*. Vol. 2. London, UK, John Libbey, 1990, pp 27–40.

Eaton S, Eaton S, Konner M: Paleolithic nutrition revisited: A twelve-year retrospective on its nature and implications. *Eur J Cl N* 1997; 51:207–216.

Eaton S, Eaton S, Sinclair A, et al: Dietary intake of long-chain polyunsaturated fatty acids during the Paleolithic. *World Rev N* 1998; 83:12–23.

Eaton S, Konner M, Shostak M: Stone agers in the fast lane: Chronic degenerative diseases in evolutionary perspective. *Am J Med* 1988;84:739–749.

Eaton S, Nelson D: Calcium in evolutionary perspective. *Am J Clin N* 1991;54:281S–287S.

Flagg E, Coates R, Calle E, et al: Correlates of red meat consumption among participants in the American Cancer Society cancer prevention study II nutrition survey. *Am J Epidem* 1996; 143:58 (meeting abstract).

Grundy S: What is the desirable ratio of saturated, polyunsaturated, and monounsaturated fatty acids in the diet? *Am J Clin N* 1997;66(suppl): 988S–990S.

Guil J, Torija M, Gimenez J, et al: Identification of fatty acids in edible wild plants by gas chromatography. *J Chromatography* 1996;719:229–235.

Gurr M: Dietary lipids and evolution of the human brain. *Br J Nutr* 1998; 79:389–390.

Hu F, Stampfer M, Rimm E, et al: A prospective study of egg consumption and risk of cardiovascular disease in men and women. *J Am Med A* 1999; 281;1387–1394.

Hunter gatherers and paleolithic nutrition. *Fd Austral* 2000;52:16.

Jin C, Yin-Chun S, Gui-Qui C, et al: Ethnobotanical studies on wild edible fruits in southern Yunnan: Folk names; Nutritional value and uses. *Econ Botan* 1999; 53:2–14.

Kleiner S: Water: An essential but overlooked nutrient. *J Am Diet A* 1999;99:200–206.

Krebs-Smith S, Cleveland L, Ballard-Barbash R, et al: Characterizing food intake patterns of American adults. *Am J Clin N* 1997; 65:1264–1268.

Krebs-Smith S, Cook D, Subar A, et al: US Adults fruit and vegetable intakes, 1989 to 1991: A revised baseline for the Healthy People 2000 objective. *Am J Pub He* 1995;85:1623–1629.

Kuhnlein H: Nutrient values in the indigenous wild plant greens and roots used by the Naxalk people of Bella Coola, British Columbia. *J Food Comp Anal* 1990;3:38–46.

Lalueza C, Perex-Perex A, Turbon D: Dietary inferences through buccal microwear analysis of middle and upper Pleistocene human fossils. *Am J P Anth* 1996;100:367–387.

Lee R: What hunters do for a living, or, how to make out on scarce resources, in Lee R, DeVore I (eds): *Man the Hunter*. Aldine, Chicago, Ill, 1968, pp 30–48.

Milton K: Hunter-gatherer diets—a different perspective. *Am J Clin N* 2000;71:665–667.

Morris E, Witkind W, Dix R, et al: Nutritional content of selected aboriginal foods in northeastern Colorado: Buffalo (Bison bison) and wild onions. *J Ethnobiol* 1981;1:213–320.

Naughton J, O'Dea K, Sinclair A: Animal foods in traditional Australian Aboriginal diets: Polyunsaturated and low in fat. *Lipids* 1986;21:684–690.

Nicklas T, Farris R, Myers L, et al: Impact of meat consumption on nutritional quality and cardiovascular risk factors in young adults: The Bogalusa Heart Study. *J Am Diet A* 1995;95:887–892.

Nicklas T, Myers L, Beech B, et al: Trends in dietary intake of sugars of 10-year-old children from 1973 to 1988: The Bogalusa Heart Study. *Nutr Res* 1999;19:519–530.

O'Dea K: Traditional diet and food preferences of Australian aboriginal hunter-gatherers. *Phil Tr R Soc L* 1991;334:233–241.

Paterson B, Block G, Rosenberger W, et al: Fruit and vegetables in the American diet: Data from the NHANES II survey. *Am J Pub He* 1990;80:1443–1449.

Redgrave T, Jeffery F: The lipids of kangaroo meat. *Lipids* 1981;16:626–627.

Schroeder H: Losses of vitamins and trace minerals resulting from processing and preservation of foods. *Am J Clin N* 1971;24:562–573.

Simopoulos A: Evolutionary aspects of omega-3 fatty acids in the food supply. *Pros Leuk E* 1999;60:421–429.

Sinclair A, O'Dea K: The significance of arachidonic acid in hunter-gatherer diets: Implications for the contemporary Western diet. *J Food Lipids* 1993;I:143–157.

Smith H, Tompkins R: Toward a life-history of the hominidae. *Am R Anthr* 1995;24:257–279.

Thorogood M, Mann J, Appleby P, et al: Risk of death from cancer and ischaemic heart disease in meat and non-meat eaters. *Br Med J* 1994;308:1667–1671.

Velasco-Vazquez J, Arnay de la Rosa M, Gonzalez-Reimers E, et al: Paleodietary analysis on the prehistoric population of El Hierro (Canary Islands). *Biol Tr El* 1997;60:235–241.

Wallace P, Marfo E, Plahar W: Nutritional quality and antinutritional composition of four non-conventional leafy vegetables. *Food Chem* 1998;61: 287–291.

Chapter 3

Ackman R: Has evolution and long-term coexistence adapted us to cope with trans fatty acids? *J Food Lipids* 1997;4:295–318.

Adams P, Lawson S, Sanigorski A, et al: Arachidonic acid to eicosapentaenoic acid ratio in blood correlates positively with clinical symptoms of depression. *Lipids* 1996;31(suppl):S157–S161.

Adlercreutz H: Evolution, nutrition, intestinal microflora, and prevention of cancer: A hypothesis. *R Soc Exp M* 1998;217:241–246.

Anderson J, Akanji A: Dietary fiber: An overview. *Diabet Care* 1991;14(12): 1126–1131.

Barnard R, Youngren J, Martin D: Diet, not aging, causes skeletal muscle insulin resistance. *Gerontology* 1995;41:205–211.

Beckman K, Ames B: The free radical theory of aging matures. *Physiol Rev* 1998;78:547–581.

Belch J, Muir A: n-6 and n-3 essential fatty acids in rheumatoid arthritis and other rheumatic conditions. *P Nutr Soc* 1998;57:563–569.

Bell L, Hectorn K, Reynolds H, et al: Cholesterol-lowering effects of soluble fiber cereals as part of a prudent diet for patients with mild to moderate hypercholesterolemia. *Am J Clin N* 1990;52:1020–1026.

Bengmark S: Ecoimmunonutrition: A challenge for the third millennium. *Nutrition* 1998;14:563–572.

Bengmark S: Ecological control of the gastrointestinal tract. The role of probiotic flora. *Gut* 1998;42:2–7.

Bengmark S: Econutrition and health maintenance: A new concept to prevent GI inflammation, ulceration, and sepsis. *Clin Nutr* 1996;15:1–10.

Bergamini E, Gori Z: Towards an understanding of the anti-aging mechanism of dietary restriction: A signal transduction theory of aging. *Aging* 1995;7:473–475.

Block G, Patterson B, Subar A: Fruit, vegetables, and cancer prevention: A review of the epidemiological evidence. *Nutr Cancer* 1992;18:1–29.

Brand J, Snow B, Nabhan G, et al: Plasma glucose and insulin responses to traditional Pima Indian meals. *Am J Clin N* 1990;51:416–420.

Breivik J, Gaudernack G: Carcinogenesis and natural selection: A new perspective to the genetics and epigenetics of colorectal cancer. *Adv Cancer R* 1999;76:187–212.

Briehl M, Baker A: Modulation of the antioxidant defense as a factor in apoptosis. *Death Diff* 1996;3:63–70.

Cao G, Booth S, Sadowski J, et al: Increases in human plasma antioxidant capacity after consumption of controlled diets high in fruit and vegetables. *Am J Clin N* 1998;68:1080–1087.

Dawson-Hughes B, Dallal G, Krall E, et al: Effect of vitamin D supplementation on wintertime and overall bone loss in healthy postmenopausal women. *Ann Int Med* 1991;115:505–512.

Fields M: Nutritional factors adversely influencing the glucose/insulin system. *J Am Col N* 1998;17:317–321.

Gibson G: Dietary modulation of the human gut microflora using prebiotics. *Br J Nutr* 1998;80:S209–S212.

Goh Y, Jumpsen J, Ryan E, et al: Effect of $w3$ fatty acid on plasma lipids, cholesterol and lipoprotein fatty acid content of NIDDM patients. *Diabetolog* 1997;40:42–52.

Goodman M, Wilkens L, Hankin J, et al: Association of soy and fiber consumption with the risk of endometrial cancer. *Am J Epidem* 1997;146:294–306.

Halliwell B: Antioxidants and human disease: A general introduction. *Nutr Rev* 1997;55:S44–S49.

Hibbeln J, Linnoila M, Umhau J, et al: Essential fatty acids predict metabolites of serotonin and dopamine in cerebrospinal fluid among healthy control subjects and early- and late-onset alcoholics. *Biol Psych* 1998;44:235–242.

Hibbeln J, Umhau J, Linnoila M, et al: A replication study of violent and nonviolent subjects: Cerebrospinal fluid metabolites of serotonin and dopamine are predicted by plasma essential fatty acids. *Biol Psych* 1998;44:243–249.

Holman R: The slow discovery of the importance of $w3$ essential fatty acids in human health. *J Nutr* 1998;128:427S–433S.

Horrobin D, Bennett C: Depression and bipolar disorders: Relationships to impaired fatty acid and phospholipid metabolism. *Pros Leuk E* 1999; 60:217–234.

Ingram D, Sanders K, Kolybaba M, et al: Case-control study of phyto-oestrogens and breast cancer. *Lancet* 1997;350:990–994.

Jacobs D, Meyer K, Kushi L, et al: Is whole grain intake associated with reduced total and cause-specific death rates in older women? The Iowa Women's Health Study. *Am J Pub He* 1999;89:322–329.

Jenkins D, Popovich D, Kendall C, et al: Effect of a diet high in vegetables, fruit, and nuts on serum lipids. *Metabolism* 1997;46:530–537.

Joseph J, Denisova N, Fisher D, et al: Age-related neurodegeneration and oxidative stress. *Neurol Aging* 1998;16:747–755.

Joseph J, Shukitt-Hale B, Denisova N, et al: Long-term dietary strawberry, spinach, or vitamin E supplementation retards the onset of age-related neuronal signal-transduction and cognitive behavioral deficits. *J Neurosc* 1998;18:8047–8055.

Keenleyside A: Skeletal evidence of health and disease in pre-contact Alaskan Eskimos and Aleuts. *Am J Anth* 1998;107:51–70.

Koppal T, Subramaniam R, Drake J, et al: Vitamin E protects against Alzheimer's amyloid peptide (25–35) induced changes in neocortical synaptosomal membrane lipid structure and composition. *Brain Res* 1998;786:270–273.

Kruger M, Coetzer H, de Winter R, et al: Calcium, gamma linolenic acid and eicosapentaenoic acid supplementation in senile osteoporosis. *Aging* 1998;10:385–394.

La Vecchia C, Decarli A, Pagano R: Vegetable consumption and risk of chronic disease. *Epidemiolog* 1998;9:208–210.

La Vecchia C, Travani A: Fruit and vegetables, and human cancer. *Eur J Can P* 1998;7:3–8.

Maes M, Christophe A, Delanghe J, et al: Lowered *w*3 polyunsaturated fatty acids in serum phospholipids and cholesterol esters of depressed patients. *Psychiat R* 1999;85:275–291.

Martin R: Docohexaenoic acid decreases phospholipase A2 activity in the neurites/nerve growth cones of PC 12 cells. *J Neurosc R* 1998;54:805–813.

Matkovic V, Ilich J: Calcium requirements for growth: Are current recommendations adequate? *Nutr Rev* 1993;51(6):171–180.

McMurry M, Cerqueira M, Connor S, et al: Changes in lipid and lipoprotein levels and body weight in Tarahumara Indians after consumption of an affluent diet. *N Eng J Med* 1991;325:1704–1708.

Means L, Higgins J, Fernandez T: Mid-life onset of dietary restriction extends life and prolongs cognitive functioning. *Physl Beh* 1993;54:503–508.

Morton M, Bundred N, McMichael-Phillips D, et al: Phyto-oestrogens and breast cancer. *Endocr-R Ca* 1997;4:331–339.

Murphy S, Khaw K, May H, et al: Milk consumption and bone mineral density in middle-aged and elderly women. *Br J Med* 1994;308:939–941.

Nagata C, Takatsuka N, Inaba S, et al: Effect of soymilk consumption on serum estrogen concentrations in premenopausal Japanese women. *J Nat Canc* 1998;90: 1830–1835.

Neel J: *Physician to the Gene Pool*. New York, Wiley, 1994, pp 302, 315, 355.

Ness A, Powles J: Fruit and vegetables, and cardiovascular disease: A review. *Int J Epid* 1997;26:1–13.

O'Dea K: Westernization, insulin resistance and diabetes in Australian aborigines. *Med J Aust* 1991;155:258–264.

Paleolithic diet, evolution, and carcinogens. *Science* 1987;238:1633–1634.

Paolisso G, Tagliamonte M, Rizzo M, et al: Oxidative stress and advancing age: Results from healthy centenarians. *J Am Ger So* 1998;46:833–838.

Reddy K, Yusuf S: Emerging epidemic of cardiovascular disease in developing countries. *Circulation* 1998;97:596–601.

Riccardi G, Rivellese A: Effects of dietary fiber and carbohydrate on glucose and lipoprotein metabolism in diabetic patients. *Diabet Care* 1991; 14(12):1115–1125.

Rimm E, Ascherio A, Giovannucci E, et al: Vegetable, fruit, and cereal fiber intake and risk of coronary heart disease among men. *J Am Med A* 1996;275:447–451.

Rimm E, Stampfer M, Ascherio A, et al: Vitamin E consumption and the risk of coronary heart disease in men. *N Eng J Med* 1993;328:1450–1456.

Salyers A, Kuritza A, McCarthy R: Influence of dietary fiber on the intestinal environment. *P Soc Exp M* 1985;180(3):415–421.

Schultz M: Meningeal diseases in infancy, from prehistory to early modern times. *Am J P Anth* 1999;S28:244.

Sies H, Stahl W: Carotenoids and intercellular communication via gap junctions. *Int J Vit N* 1997;67:364–367.

Sinclair A: Was the hunter-gatherer diet prothrombotic? In Sinclair A, Gibson R (eds): *Essential Fatty Acids and Eicosanoids.* Champaign, Ill, American Oil Chemists Society, 1992, pp 318–324.

Singh R, Niaz M, Ghosh S: Effect on central obesity and associated disturbances of low-energy, fruit- and vegetable-enriched prudent diet in North Indians. *Postg Med J* 1994;70:895–900.

Steinmetz K, Childs M, Stimson C, et al: Effect of consumption of whole milk and skim milk on blood lipid profiles in healthy men. *Am J Clin N* 1994;59:612–618.

Taylor G, Williams C: Effects of probiotics and prebiotics on blood lipids. *Br J Nutr* 1998;80:S225–S230.

Troisi R, Willett W, Weiss S: Trans fatty acid intake in relation to serum lipid concentrations in adult men. *Am J Clin N* 1992; 56: 1019–1024.

Troyer D, Fernandes G: Nutrition and apoptosis. *Nutr Res* 1996;16:1959–1987.

Tucker K, Hannan M, Chen H, et al: Potassium, magnesium, and fruit and vegetable intakes are associated with greater bone mineral density in elderly men and women. *Am J Clin N* 1999;69:727–736.

Vatassery G: Vitamin E and other endogenous antioxidants in the central nervous system. *Geriatrics* 1998;53:S25–S27.

Wang C, Kurzer M: Effects of phytoestrogens on DNA synthesis in MCF-7 cells in the presence of estradiol or growth factors. *Nutr Cancer* 1998;31:90–100.

Wierik E, van den Berg H: Energy restriction, the basis for successful aging in man? *Nutr Res* 1994;14:1113–1134.

Willett W, Ascherio A: Trans fatty acids: Are the effects only marginal? *Am J Pub He* 1994;84:722–724.

Williams D, Wareham N, Cox B, et al: Frequent salad vegetable consumption is associated with a reduction in the risk of diabetes mellitus. *J Clin Epid* 1999;52:329–335.

Worthington V: Effect of agricultural methods on nutritional quality: A comparison of organic with conventional crops. *Altern Ther* 1998;4:58–69.

Yamasaki H, Omori Y, Zaidan-Dagli M, et al: Genetic and epigenetic changes of intercellular communication genes during multistage carcinogenesis. *Cancer Det* 1999;23:273–279.

Yehuda S, Rabinovitz S, Mostofsky D: Essential fatty acids are mediators of brain biochemistry and cognitive functions. *J Neurosc R* 1999;56:565–570.

Zhang J, Sasaki S, Amano K, et al: Fish consumption and mortality from all causes, ischemic heart disease, and stroke: An ecological study. *Prev Med* 1999;28:520–529.

Chapter 4

Andersen R, Crespo C, Bartlett S, et al: Relationship of physical activity and television watching with body weight and level of fatness among children. *J Am Med A* 1998;279:938–942.

Bell E, Castellanos V, Pelkman C, et al: Energy density of foods affects energy intake in normal-weight women. *Am J Clin N* 1998;67:412–420.

Bindon J, Baker P: Bergmann's Rule and the Thrifty Genotype. *Am J P Anth* 1997;104:201–210.

Blundell J, Macdiarmid J: Passive overconsumption: Fat intake and short-term energy balance. *Ann NY Acad* 1997;827:392–407.

Blundell J, Stubbs R: High and low carbohydrate and fat intakes: Limits imposed by appetite and palatability and their implications for energy balance. *Eur J Cl N* 1999;53:S148–S165.

Burrows E, Henry H, Bowen D, et al: Nutritional applications of a clinical low fat dietary intervention to public health change. *J Nutr Ed* 1993;25:167–175.

Cordain L, Gotshall R, Eaton S: Evolutionary aspects of exercise. *World Rev. N* 1997;81:49–60.

Cotton J, Burley V, Weststrate J, et al: Dietary fat and appetite: Similarities and differences in the satiating effect of meals supplemented with either fat or carbohydrate. *J Hum Nu Di* 1994;7:11–24.

DeCastro J, Brewer E, Elmore D, et al: Social facilitation of the spontaneous meal size of humans occurs regardless of time, place, alcohol, and snacks. *Appetite* 1990;15:89–101.

Deheeger M, Rolland-Cachera M, Fontvielle A: Physical activity and body composition in 10-year-old French children: Linkages with nutritional intake. *Int J Obes* 1997;21:372–379.

Eaton S, Cordain L: Evolutionary aspects of diet: Old genes, new fuels. *World Rev N* 1997;81:26–37.

Feunekes G, DeGraaf C, Van Staveren W: Social facilitation of food intake is mediated by meal duration. *Physl Behav* 1995;58:551–559.

Galef B: Food selection: Problems in understanding how we choose foods to eat. *Neurosci B* 1996;20:67–73.

Geiselman P: Control of food intake. *End Metab C* 1996;25:815–829.

Harnack L, Story M, Rock B: Diet and physical activity patterns of Lakota Indian adults. *J Am Diet A* 1999;99:829–835.

Hart R, Turturro A: Evolution and dietary restriction. *Exp Geront* 1998;33:53–60.

Heitmann B, Lissner L, Sorensen T, et al: Dietary fat intake and weight gain in women genetically predisposed for obesity. *Am J Clin N* 1995;61:1213–1217.

Hill J, Peters J: Environmental contributors to the obesity epidemic. *Science* 1998;280:1371–1374.

Himaya A, Louis-Sylvestre J: The effect of soup on satiation. *Appetite* 1998;30:199–210.

Kuzawa C: Adipose tissue in human infancy and childhood: An evolutionary perspective. *Yearbook of Physical Anthropology* 1998;41:177–209.

Lands W: Alcohol, calories, and appetite. *Vitam Horm* 1998;54:31–49.

Lappalainen R, Mennen L, van Weert L, et al: Drinking water with a meal: A simple method of coping with feelings of hunger, satiety, and desire to eat. *Eur J Clin N* 1993;47:815–819.

Lawton C, Burley V, Wales J, et al: Dietary fat and appetite control in obese subjects: Weak effects on satiation and satiety. *Int J Obes* 1993;17:409–416.

Leibowitz S, Akabayashi A, Wang J: Obesity on a high-fat diet: Role of hypothalamic galanin in neurons of the anterior paraventricular nucleus projecting to the median eminence. *J Neurosc* 1998;18:2709–2719.

Miller G, Groziak S: Impact of fat substitutes on fat intake. *Lipids* 1996;31:S293–S296.

Oygard L, Klepp K: Influences of social groups on eating patterns: A study among young adults. *J Behav Med* 1996;19:1.

Phillipson C: Paleonutrition and modern nutrition. *World Rev N* 1997;81:38–48.

Popkin B. Udry J: Adolescent obesity increases significantly in second and third generation US immigrants: The National Longitudinal Study of Adolescent Health. *J Nutr* 1998;128:701–706.

Poston W, Foreyt J: Obesity is an environmental issue. *Atheroscler* 1999;146:201–209.

Rolls B: Sensory-specific satiety. *Nutr Rev* 1986;44:93–101.

Rolls B, Kim-Harris S, Fischman M, et al: Satiety after preloads with different amounts of fat and carbohydrate: Implications for obesity. *Am J Clin N* 1994;60:476–487.

Speth J: Early hominid hunting and scavenging: The role of meat as an energy source. *J Hum Evol* 1989;18:329–343.

Tiwary C, Ward J, Jackson B: Effect of pectin on satiety in healthy US army adults. *J Am Col N* 19997;16:423–428.

Chapter 5

Burton G, Traber M, Acuff R, et al: Human plasma and tissue alpha tocopherol concentrations in response to supplementation with deuterated natural and synthetic vitamin E. *Am J Clin N* 1998;67:669–684.

Chatenoud L, Tavani A, LaVecchia C, et al: Whole grain food intake and cancer risk. *Int J Canc* 1998;77:24–28.

Coulston A: Limitations on the adage "eat a variety of foods"? *Am J Clin N* 1999;69:350–351.

Donovan U, Gibson R: Dietary intakes of adolescent females consuming vegetarian, semi-vegetarian, and omnivorous diets. *J Adoles H* 1996;18:292–300.

Dreher M, Maher C, Kearney P: The traditional and emerging role of nuts in healthful diets. *Nutr Rev* 1996;54:241–245.

Favell D: A comparison of the vitamin C content of fresh and frozen vegetables. *Food Chem* 1998;62:59–64.

Hackett A, Nathan I, Burgess L: Is a vegetarian diet adequate for children? *Nutr Health* 1998;12:189–195.

Hu J, Zhao X, Jia J, et al: Dietary calcium and bone density among middle-aged and elderly women in China. *Am J Clin N* 1993;58:219–227.

Jacobs D, Marquart L, Slavin J, et al: Whole-grain intake and cancer: An expanded review and meta-analysis. *Nutr Cancer* 1998;30:85–96.

Jacobs D, Meyer K, Kushi L, et al: Is whole grain intake associated with reduced total and cause-specific death rates in older women? The Iowa Women's Health Study. *Am J Pub He* 1999;89:322–329.

Jacobs D, Slavin J, Marquart L: Whole grain intake and cancer: A review of the literature. *Nutr Cancer* 1995;24:221–229.

Key T, Thorogood M, Appleby P, et al: Dietary habits and mortality in 11,000 vegetarians and health conscious people: Results of a 17-year follow up. *Br Med J* 1996;313:775–779.

Margetts B, Beilin L, Vandongen R, et al: Vegetarian diet in mild hypertension: A randomized controlled trial. *Br Med J* 1986;293:1468–1471.

Munoz K, Krebs-Smith S, Ballard-Barbash R, et al: Food intakes of US children and adolescents compared with recommendations. *Pediatrics* 1997;100:323–329.

Murphy S, Khaw K, May H, et al: Milk consumption and bone mineral density in middle-aged and elderly women. *Br Med J* 1994;308:939–941.

Newsome W, Davies D, Sun W: Residues of polychlorinated biphenyls (PCBs) in fatty foods of the Canadian diet. *Food Addit* 1998;15:19–29.

Oakley G, Adams M, Dickenson C: More folic acid for everyone, now. *J Nutr* 1996;126:S751–S755.

Ranhotra G, Gelroth J, Novak F, et al: Nutritive value of selected variety breads and pastas. *J Am Diet A* 1984;84:322–327.

Shearer M. Bach A, Kohlmeier M: Chemistry, nutritional sources, a tissue distribution and metabolism of vitamin K with special reference to bone health. *J Nutr* 1996;126:1181S–1186S.

Singh R, Niaz M, Ghosh S, et al: Effect of central obesity and associated disturbances of low-energy, fruit- and vegetable-enriched prudent diet in North Indians. *Postg Med J* 1994;70:895–900.

Slavin J, Jacobs D, Marquart L: Whole-grain consumption and chronic disease: Protective mechanisms. *Nutr Cancer* 1997;27:14–21.

Snowdown D, Phillips R, Fraser G: Meat consumption and fatal ischemic heart disease. *Prev Med* 1984;13:490–500.

Thorogood M, Mann J, Appleby P, et al: Risk of death from cancer and ischemic heart disease in meat and non-meat eaters. *Br Med J* 1994;308:1667–1671.

Ullmann D, Connor W, Hatcher L, et al: Will a high-carbohydrate, low-fat diet lower plasma lipids and lipoproteins without producing hypertriglyceridemia? *Arter Throm* 1991;11:1059–1067.

Verma S, Goldin B: Effect of soy-derived isoflavonoids on the induced growth of MCF-7 by estrogenic environmental chemicals. *Cancer* 1998;30:232–239.

Warman P, Havard K: Yield, vitamin and minerals contents of organically and conventionally grown potatoes and sweet corn. *Agri Eco E* 1998;68:207–216.

Chapter 6

Anderson R, Wadden T, Barlett S, et al: Effects of lifestyle activity vs structured aerobic exercise in obese women. *J Am Med A* 1999;281:335–340.

Caspersen C, Merritt R: Physical activity trends among 26 states, 1986–1990. *Med Sci Spt* 1995;27:713–720.

Christensen H, Mackinnon A: The association between mental, social and physical activity and cognitive performance in young and old subjects. *Age Aging* 1993;22:175–182.

Corcoran P: Use it or lose it: The hazards of bed rest and inactivity. *West J Med* 1991;154:536–538.

Cordain L, Gotshall R, Eaton S: Evolutionary aspects of exercise. *World Rev N* (Karger) 1997;81:49–60.

Coyle C, Santiago M: Aerobic exercise training and depressive symptomatology in adults with physical disabilities. *Arch Phys M* 1995;76:647–652.

Dunn A, Andersen R, Jakicic J: Lifestyle physical activity interventions. History, short- and long-term effects, and recommendations. *Am J Prev M* 1998; 15:398–412.

Dunn A, Marcus H, Kampert B, et al: Comparison of lifestyle and structured interventions to increase physical activity and cardiovascular fitness. *J Am Med A* 1999;281:327–334.

Evans W: Reversing sarcopenia: How weight training can build strength and vitality. *Geriatrics* 1996;51:46–53.

Giada F, Vigna G, Vitale E, et al: Effect of age on the response of blood lipids, body composition, and aerobic power to physical conditioning and decon-ditioning. *Metabolism* 1995;44:161–165.

Hayes D, Ross C: Body and mind: The effect of exercise, overweight, and phys-ical health on psychological well-being. *J Health So* 1986;27:387–400.

Heitkamp H, Schmid K, Scheib K: Beta endorphin and adrenocorticotropic hormone production during marathon and incremental exercise. *Eur J A Phy* 1993;66:269–274.

Lee I, Hsieh C, Paffenbarger R: Exercise intensity and longevity in men: The Harvard Alumni Health Study. *J Am Med A* 1995;273:1179–1184.

Owens J, Matthews K, Wing R, et al: Can physical activity mitigate the effects of aging in middle-aged women? *Circulation* 1992;85:1265–1270.

Paolisso G, Gambardella A, Balbi V, et al: Body composition, body fat distribu-tion, and resting metabolic rate in healthy centenarians. *Am J Clin N* 1995;62:746–750.

Pate R, Pratt M, Blair S, et al: Physical activity and public health: A recommen-dation from the Centers for Disease Control and Prevention and the Amer-ican College of Sports Medicine. *J Am Med A* 1995;273:402–407.

Pierce E, Eastman N, Tripathi H, et al: Beta endorphin response to endurance exercise: Relationship to exercise dependence. *Perc Mot Sk* 1993;77:767–770.

Pratt M: Benefits of lifestyle activity vs structured exercise. *J Am Med A* 1999;281:375—376.

Schwarz L, Kindermann W: Changes in beta endorphin levels in response to aerobic and anaerobic exercise. *Sport Med* 1992;13:25—36.

Shellock F: Physiological benefits of warm-up. *Phys Sport* 1983;11:134—139.

Shephard R, Balady G: Exercise as cardiovascular therapy. *Circulation* 1999;99:963—972.

Silverman H, Mazzeo R: Hormonal responses to maximal and submaximal exercise in trained and untrained men of various ages. *J Gerontol* 1996; 51A: B30—B37.

Stillman R, Lohman T, Slaughter M, et al: Physical activity and bone mineral content in women aged 30 to 85 years. *Med Sci Spt* 1986;18:576—580.

Williams T, Krahenbuhl G, Morgan D: Mood state and running economy in moderately trained male runners. *Med Sci Spt* 1991;23:727—731.

Chapter 7

Burchfield S, Holmes T, Harrington R: Personality differences between sick and rarely sick individuals. *Soc Sci Med* 1981;15E:145—148.

Cassel J: An epidemiological perspective of psychosocial factors in disease etiology. *Am J Pub He* 1974;64:1040—1043.

Chew F, Goh D, Ooi B, et al: Association of ambient air-pollution levels with acute asthma exacerbation among children in Singapore. *Allergy* 1999;54: 320—329.

Chrousos G, Gold P: The concepts of stress and stress system disorders. *J Am Med A* 1992; 267: 1244—1252.

Cobb S: Social support as a moderator of life stress. *Psychosom Med* 1976;38:300—313.

Duclos M, Corcuff J, Etcheverry N, et al: Abdominal obesity increases overnight cortisol excretion. *J Endoc Inv* 1999;22:465—471.

Edge-Gumble S: Flower power. *Health-Facil Mug* 1996; 9: 20—26, 28.

Fairley D: Daily mortality and air pollution in Santa Clara County, California: 1989—1996. *Envir Hlth Persp* 1999;107:637—641.

Feher S, Maly R: Coping with breast cancer in later life: The role of religious faith. *Psychooncology* 1999;8:408—416.

Foley R: The adaptive legacy of human evolution: A search for the environment of evolutionary adaptedness. *Evol Anthr* 1995;4:194—203.

Herbert T, Cohen S: Stress and immunity in humans: A meta-analytic review. *Psychosom Med* 1993;55:364—379.

Jabaau L, Grosheide P, Heijtink R, et al: Influence of perceived psychological stress and distress on antibody response to low dose rDNA hepatitis B vaccine. *J Psychosom R* 1993;37:361–369.

Jamriska M, Thomas S, Morawska L, et al: Relation between indoor and outdoor exposure to fine particles near a busy arterial road. *Indoor Air* 1999;9:75–84.

Jayo J, Shively C, Kaplan J, et al: Effects of exercise and stress on body fat distribution in male cynomolgus monkeys. *Int J Obes* 1993;17:597–604.

Jennison K: The impact of stressful life events and social support on drinking among older adults: A general population survey. *Int J Agin Hu Dev* 1992;35:99–123.

Kash K, Holland J, Halper M, et al: Psychological distress and surveillance behaviors of women with a family history of breast cancer. *JNCI* 1992;84:24–30.

Kelly S, Hertzman C, Daniels M: Searching for the biological pathways between stress and health. *Ann R Pub H* 1997;18:437–462.

Lao Y, Smith R, Rich T, et al: Carbon monoxide levels in homes with fuel-burning space heaters. *J Environ Health* 1982;44:180–182.

Lee J, Shin D, Chung Y: Air pollution and daily mortality in Seoul and Ulsan, Korea. *Environ Health Perspect* 1999;107:149–154.

Le Fur C, Romon M, Lebel P, et al: Influence of mental stress and circadian cycle on postprandial lipidemia. *Am J Clin N* 1999;70:213–220.

Leger D: The cost of sleep-related accidents: A report for the National Commission on Sleep Disorders Research. *Sleep* 1994;17:84–93.

Lemus R, Abdelghani A, Akers T, et al: Potential health risks from exposure to formaldehyde. *Rev Environ Health* 1998;13:91–98.

Marks I, Nesse R: Fear and fitness: An evolutionary analysis of anxiety disorders. *Ethology and Sociobiology* 1994;15:247–261.

Maslow A: *Toward a Psychology of Being.* New York, D. Van Nostrand Company, 1968.

McWeen B, Stellar E: Stress and the individual: Mechanisms leading to disease. *Arch In Med* 1993;153:2093–2101.

Meggs W: Health effects of indoor air pollution. *NCMJ* 1992;53:354–357.

Oliver L, Shackleton B: The indoor air we breathe. *Public Health Rep* 1998;113:398–409.

Posner I, Leitner L, Lester D: Diet, cigarette smoking, stressful life events, and subjective feelings of stress. *Psychol Rep* 1994;74:841–842.

Schleifer S, Keller S, Stein M: Stress effects on immunity. *Psychiat J U Ottawa* 1985;10:125–131.

Schwartz J: Air pollution and daily mortality in Birmingham, Alabama. *Am J Epidem* 1993; 137:1136–1147.

Seelig M, Master A: Consequences of magnesium deficiency on the enhancement of stress reactions: Preventive and therapeutic implications. *J Am Col N* 1994;13:429–446.

Singh A, Smoak B, Patterson K, et al: Biochemical indices of selected trace minerals in men: Effect of stress. *Am J Clin N* 1991;53:126–131.

Snyder B, Roghmann K, Sigal L: Stress and psychosocial factors: Effects on primary cellular immune response. *J Behav Med* 1993;16:143–160.

Spiegel D, Bloom J, Kraemer H, et al: Effect of psychosocial treatment on survival of patients with metastatic breast cancer. *Lancet* 1989;ii:888–91.

Stenberg B, Eriksson N, Hoog J, et al: The sick building syndrome (SBS) in office workers. A case-referent study of personal, psychosocial and building-related risk indicators. *Int J Epidem* 1994;23:1190–1197.

Stone A, Boybjerg D, Neale J, et al: Development of common cold symptoms following experimental rhinovirus infection is related to prior stressful life events. *Behav Med* 1992;18:115–120.

Uchino B, Holt-Lunstad J, Uno D, et al: Social support and age-related differences in cardiovascular function: An examination of potential mediators. *Ann Behav Med* 1992;21:135–142.

Vandervoort D: Quality of social support in mental and physical health. *Curr Psych* 1999;18:205–221.

Wargocki P, Wyon D, Baik Y, et al: Perceived air quality, sick building syndrome symptoms and productivity in an office with two different pollution loads. *Indoor Air* 1999;9:165–179.

Wetter D, Young T: The relation between cigarette smoking and sleep disturbance. *Prev Med* 1994;23:328–334.

Wildassin S: Fresh air, sunshine, flowers combat doldrums, aid in rehabilitation. *Volunt Leader* 1980;21:14.

Williams R, Barefoot J, Califf R, et al: Prognostic importance of social and economic resources among medically treated patients with angiographically documented coronary artery disease. *J Am Med A* 1992;267:520–524.

Zmirou D, Deloraine A, Balducci F, et al: Health effects costs of particulate air pollution. *J Occ Env Med* 1999;41:847–856.

Index

Index

Index

Index

Index

Index

Index

vegan diets, 164
vegetable oils, 46
  hydrogenating, 49–50, 148
vegetables, 16, 38, 39, 56, 57, 60, 109, 111, 137,
    138, 163, 164, 223
  adding servings of, 135–36
  anti-cancer army in, 71–72
  benefits from, 69–70, 165
  dark green leafy, 39, 40, 84
  fresh, frozen, canned, 136–37
  lower cancer risk, xiv
  nutrient-dense, 39–40
  in Origin Diet, 127, 132, 134–39
  in Origin Pyramid, 125
  phytochemicals in, 71
  recipes, 274–78
  starchy, 149
vegetarian diets, 22
  evolution and, 163–64
vitamin A, 4, 13, 40
  deficiency, 23
vitamin B$_1$, 40
vitamin B$_2$, 39, 164
vitamin B$_6$, 67, 82, 164, 198
vitamin B$_{12}$, 164, 165
vitamin C, 4, 39, 40, 65, 67, 132, 136, 164, 198
  deficiency, 23
  sources of, 59, 124
vitamin D, 21, 40, 54, 67, 81, 84–85, 164–65
  deficiency, 15, 84–85
  sources of, 154
  supplements, 155
vitamin deficiency, 13, 198, 206
vitamin E, 6, 40, 54, 65, 67, 91, 164
  supplements, 167
vitamin K, 88, 165
vitamins, 21, 164
  added to food, 58, 59
  in fruits and vegetables, 39–40, 136–37
  in organic produce, 138

Wadden, Thomas, 105, 115, 183–84
walking, 24, 93, 179, 182
  ancient ancestors, 170–72, 173
  stress reduction through, 186–87
water, 31, 38, 54–55, 60, 107, 113, 144–46, 223
  in Origin Diet, 128
Watkins, Bruce, 80–81
waxes, 137–38
weight, 22, 38, 39
  physical activity and, 49

weight gain, xiv, 96–101, 107, 128
  risk for, 62
  sleep deprivation and, 204
weight lifting, 24, 189–90, 194
weight loss, xvi, xvii, 63, 69, 106–7, 109–10
  body's defenses against, 107, 108f
  with daily activity, 183–84
  evolutionary, 95–120
  water in, 145
weight maintenance, 60, 175
weight management, 163
  guidelines, 110–20
westernized societies
  diseases in, 61–62, 68–69
  high-protein diets, 50
  and obesity, 97
wheat germ, 151
whole grains, 44, 57, 60, 73, 75, 109, 111, 125,
    137, 164
  benefits from, 165
  and disease risk, 163
  in Origin Diet, 127, 149–51
  variety in, 132
wild (natural) foods, 24
wild game, 7, 12, 24, 32, 34, 36, 39, 44–45, 58,
    60
  cholesterol in, 49
  fat in, 45–46, 79
  hunted to extinction, 11
  modern-day hunter-gatherers and, 35
  nutritional analysis of, 33, 37
  nutritionally different from domesticated meat,
    47t
  in Origin Diet, 127, 139–41
  sources of, 289
wild plants, 34, 40
  carbohydrates from, 44
Willett, Walter, 83, 149
women, 7
  calcium needs/intake, 84, 154
  daily activity, 183
  differences from men, 218–19
  nutritional status of, 14
  storing fat, 100
  supplements for, 169
  working, 207
worry, 199, 200

yogurt, 86, 88, 108

zinc, 40, 67, 164, 198

About the Author

ELIZABETH SOMER, M.A., R.D., is a nationally recognized nutrition expert and award-winning writer. She is a former monthly contributor to ABC's *Good Morning America* and NBC's *Later Today*, a contributing editor to *Shape* magazine, and editor-in-chief of the newsletter *Nutrition Alert*. The author of six books, she lives in Salem, Oregon. Her Web site can be found at www.elizabethsomer.com.